TRANSFORMATION THROUGH MENOPAUSE

TRANSFORMATION THROUGH MENOPAUSE

MARIAN VAN EYK McCAIN

BERGIN & GARVEY
New York • Westport, Connecticut • London

Library of Congress Cataloging-in-Publication Data

McCain, Marian Van Eyk.
    Transformation through menopause / Marian Van Eyk
McCain.
        p.   cm.
    Includes bibliographical references and index.
    ISBN 0–89789–268–2 (hb : alk. paper).—ISBN 0–89789–269–0
(pbk. : alk. paper)
        1. Menopause. 2. Menopause—Psychological aspects.
        I. Title.
    RG186.M35   1991
    612.6'65'019—dc20   91–12685

British Library Cataloguing in Publication Data is available.

Library of Congress Catalog Card Number: 91–12685
ISBN: 0–89789–268–2 (hb)
       0–89789–269–0 (pbk.)

First published in 1991

Bergin & Garvey, One Madison Avenue, New York, NY 10010
An imprint of Greenwood Publishing Group, Inc.

Printed in the United States of America

(∞)™

The paper used in this book complies with the
Permanent Paper Standard issued by the National
Information Standards Organization (Z39.48–1984).

10 9 8 7 6 5 4 3 2 1

To my younger sisters,
Sue and Leticia,
and all their contemporaries—
for they are the next in line.

CONTENTS

PREFACE

It seems a pity to have a built-in rite of passage and to dodge
it, evade it, and pretend nothing has changed. That is to dodge
and evade one's womanhood, to pretend one's like a man. Men,
once initiated, never get the second chance. They never change
again. That's their loss, not ours. Why borrow poverty?
                    Ursula LeGuin, "The Space Crone"

When I was a child, menopause was usually referred to as
"the change of life." The more I think of that, the more it
seems to me a far better term than "menopause" to describe
this important life phase.

Life has indeed changed, for me. It has changed in ways I
could not even have imagined a few years ago. The change is
fascinating. I never dreamed there could be so much richness
in it.

When I first began to think of menopause as a rite of passage,
it seemed like an original thought. At that stage, I had never
heard it referred to in that way; nor had I read of such a
definition. The idea came from within me, as though from
some long-forgotten knowledge, and burst into my waking
consciousness like a meteor, trailing ideas and insights as it
flashed across my mind.

It was with some trepidation that I first began mentioning
this notion to others. Even to speak of menopause seemed

slightly embarrassing to me way back then. I wondered if they would think me ridiculous.

Looking back now, at those early beginnings, I can scarcely believe that that was me. However, it was. That younger self, the one who plunged on through embarrassment, and began to express ideas, thoughts, feelings, and dreams, was the same person who set this whole book in motion. The "me of today" is grateful to the "me of yesterday," who dared to take a risk.

As I talked more to others about my ideas concerning menopause and learned to reveal my own inner experience of the "change of life" without shame or embarrassment, more was revealed to me. I discovered other women who were exploring the same paths, thinking the same thoughts, and feeling the same feelings. Furthermore, I discovered writings that gave form and voice to the inchoate messages within.

Without the validation that came from discovering shared experience, I would not have had the courage to begin my own writing. It is therefore to those others, in whose responses I heard my first echoes, that I must now give thanks.

There are some whose names I never knew, or have forgotten, although my conversations with them planted seeds which later grew in my work. I give my thanks to all those nameless ones.

Then there are those who I can acknowledge by name. My thanks go to Mary Wayne, with whom I picnicked in Golden Gate Park the day this book was first conceived, and who became a gold mine of useful ideas and information. Thanks, too, to Ofer Zur, Arlene Mazak, and Marilyn Nagy, without whose assistance the original research could never have been carried out. Thanks to Olive Elliott, who was the first person ever to ask me questions about menopause, and to Aurelio Farrugia, who was the first to see this book in my stars.

In those early days, when I was still timidly finding my beginning place, there were some little tokens of encouragement that made all the difference. I remember with gratitude the "Big Wave" postcard that arrived one morning from Dominie Cappadonna in Hawaii, expressing support just when I was feeling faint-hearted, and the enthusiastic burst of photocopying from Christine Cameron in Geelong, Australia, who used her own stamps to send out letters on my behalf. Lots of small things like this were so important in their way, giving me the courage to keep talking, reading, asking, exploring— and finally, writing.

My gratitude goes out to all the women who have taken part in my research, many of whom appear in the pages of this book, their names altered to preserve their anonymity. I thank them for their courage in revealing their experiences and feelings, and for taking the time to share them with me.

Special thanks must go to all those mentors and teachers who have guided me by their word and example and by their very being. Angeles Arrien, who taught me the importance of myth and symbol, Tanya Wilkinson and Peter O'Connor, whose interpretations of Jungian psychology brought it alive with meaning, Jean Klein, who taught me the true nature of reality, and, above all, Richard Moss, who showed me how to find the doorway of experience and to enter it, and in so doing changed my life forever.

As I look up at my crowded bookshelves, I know there is no way to thank all the hundreds of people, living and dead, who have inspired and taught me through the written word. Suffice it to say that without them I would not be writing now, in my turn.

I have also gained inspiration from a small group of women whose way of living in their female bodies seems to me to epitomize the "new woman" who is gradually emerging in our culture. I carry their pictures in my mind: Mary Rizely, who led me blindfolded up a mountain path, Janina Papas, who told me to take off my make-up, and Lucy Joss, who forced me to confront my inner judgments.

Finally, I wish to thank those who have helped me in practical ways to bring this book to completion. First, Sophy Craze, and the team at Bergin and Garvey, who waited patiently for the manuscript while I was travelling in Europe and Asia, gestating it as I went. Then Jillianne Charalambous, who reinspired me, and Annette Robins, whose loyalty and encouragement remained constant and heartwarming, and who kept me thinking and writing. Thanks also to Jennifer Suich, who took time to share her ideas on lesbian women's experiences, and to the "Golden Oldies" group, who responded to my letters so willingly.

Thanks to Johanna van Eijk for her assistance with typing and with my learning process, and to Don McCain, my patient and loving partner, who has lived with this book—and with my menopause—as long as I have, and who has never flagged in his support and caring. Together, we have learned a great deal.

This book, like menopause itself, has been a rite of passage—a ritual journey into a new place from which there is no going back. I am so glad that I am me, here, now, fifty-four and fully alive.

INTRODUCTION: THE INWARD SPIRAL

Inspiration sometimes comes from unlikely sources. Who would ever have suspected that my inspiration for a book about menopause would come from such an unlikely source as Susan? Yet it did. So first I must tell you about Susan.

Susan was a child I once knew. A tall, spindly seven-year-old, with long, brown limbs and huge dark eyes that stared out into the depths of space. That is how I picture her now. Maybe memory has distorted reality, but inasmuch as Susan lives in me, this is how she lives.

She liked to sing to herself—snatches of song she had heard the other children sing—and to rock her lean body to and fro in the chair. Susan was profoundly autistic, cut off from communication. Yet in a way she did communicate. She liked to be held, and would nestle into my lap, surprisingly quiet. In the nine months that I had daily care of Susan, I struggled to know her, to see into her strange and isolated world, but I never felt we did more than begin.

There were times, too, when I felt repulsion. The epileptic seizures, the frothing mouth, the uncontrolled bladder, these made her a strange, wild animal to my eyes. Her body always wore bruises, reminders of her frequent falling, banging, crashing into things on her way down to her brief oblivion on the floor.

Thirty-five years have passed and I can still see that oddly

lanky little body with its bruises, and the way she loved to
hold a pencil and draw, endlessly repeating the same pattern.
In pencil, crayon, chalk, anything that was to hand, Susan
always drew the same thing, over and over again. It was an
inward-turning spiral, which began as a circle, speeding up
as her hand moved toward the center.

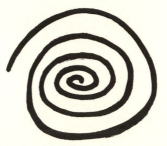

When she reached the center, she would stop. Then she would
lift her pencil and start again, somewhere else. Sheet after
sheet she would cover with these little whorls. Her signature.
Her only written statement to the world. Maybe the symbolic
cry of a tiny soul trapped deep in the center of a life she could
not comprehend—who knows?

To me, as I was then, young, strong, and thrusting outward
into the world, that inward spiral seemed like a sick place. A
dark, lonely, sick place that spoke only of isolation and despair. I could only perceive it as Susan's entrapment in her
lonely, autistic world—her dark, spiraling path to nowhere.
While the other children, growing daily in knowledge and
achievement, drew houses and people, birds and butterflies and
skies with shining suns in them, Susan turned ever inward
into herself, locked in her spiral pattern that seemed to lead
only to an inner tomb. I was repulsed by it, and my repulsion
fought with my compassion and my yearning to understand
and to touch her, to make contact with her where she lived,
to *know*.

Then it mattered less, for I had things to do. As the years
passed, the memory of Susan and her spirals lay very deeply
in the earth of my being like a patient seed. I was too busy

going somewhere. That is as it should be. Seeds need time in the dark earth.

How we have relished the straight line, the soaring graph, the ladder to the sky. Gross National Product, economic growth, development, personal growth, spiritual growth, any kind of growth, no matter what, as long as it is onward and upward like a flower. Then the flower dies and falls and we say, "What a shame," and look for another. We never watch it fall the way we watched it grow. Once past its prime, it is finished, forgotten, its usefulness gone. Time to replace it.

All our favorite metaphors for growth seem to be like that—linear. Mine certainly were. Until I too, like the flower, reached my "prime." Unlike the flower, which probably does not wonder, I wondered what lay *beyond* "prime time."

My first reaction to this wondering was to plan to extend prime time indefinitely. That is easy to do in our society. People, especially women, have been reacting that way for a long time now. I set to work to ensure that my life was full and fascinating, my body supple, slim, strong, and healthy, and my lifestyle a model of enviable wellness. I determined to live to 100, and ate the diet of Hunzas, Himalayans known for their longevity, to ensure that I would. Yoga, exercise, postgraduate studies, travel, personal growth, spiritual awakening, you name it, I was there, not only doing it but teaching others how to do it also; modeling wellness, teaching wellness, writing about wellness. And, of course, modeling humility, too, just in case anyone should think that my ego was in any way involved with all of that! That, too, was as it should be. We learn our lessons in a certain order.

The crunch comes to different people in different ways, but for me the crunch was menopause. Menopause unglued me. Menopause, and the events that coincided with it in my life, melted away every self-image, every model, every vision of who I thought I was and left me with nothing. Nothing, that is, except the sweet, light, wonderful promise of infinity.

This book is about that transformational process and how I think it works.

With my struggle to understand the workings of this process

so that I could share it, the long-buried seed of Susan's symbolism began to germinate. I found myself drawing her pattern. I found myself being pulled, as though by some new, centripetal force, into an inward-turning spiral of my own.

I knew what was happening to me on a physical level, but mentally, emotionally, and spiritually I felt confused and tortured at times. Not always, just on the dark days. There were many dark days at first, until I began to explore the process and to learn to flow with it instead of contracting against it in fear. I felt an urgent need to understand the new feelings I was having. They were like premenstrual syndrome (PMS) in some ways—and that was a familiar-enough syndrome for me—yet they had no regular, predictable rhythm. Rather they seemed random and unsettlingly frequent. Feelings of confusion, of rage, of fear; feelings of inadequacy, sadness, and doubt. All these, and more, were the feelings that now seemed to besiege me.

I worked hard to process them. Sometimes bits of understanding came from dreams. Sometimes nothing came and I found myself bogged down in confusion and depression. At those times, I began to act out my fears and feelings in a number of experimental ways. I began to try singing them or dancing them, and frequently I picked up crayons and drew them. That was when I noticed that I was often drawing Susan's spiral pattern.

I felt, like Susan, autistic. Trapped in my own, inward-turning world, I found I could no longer explain my feelings adequately to those around me. The center of the spiral seemed, once again, like a sick place, my own sick place, where all my own unresolved issues still lay. I resisted it, yet it seemed to pull me. This experience of being pulled into the center of a spiral was so strong that it began to feel as though I were on the edge of some perilous vortex, some whirlpool which would suck me down to destruction. I feared that if I reached the center, I would surely drown. I felt the same mixture of feelings toward myself as I had felt toward Susan—compassion combined with repulsion.

Some days it would be palpably physical. Fatigue, such as I had never experienced before, would overcome me and I would lie down in the middle of the afternoon. There would be a strange, fuzzy mental sensation and sometimes feelings of vertigo. Closing my eyes, I would let myself go into the feeling. My thoughts would start to spin out of control. A whirling craziness would seem to envelop me, becoming stronger and stronger, crazier and crazier. Eventually, I would drift into sleep. Half an hour or so later, I would awake with a sort of "ping" and feel refreshed and light.

At first the experience frightened me, but as I grew accustomed to it, it began to feel comforting. I realized that at the center of my spiral was not a deadly vortex after all, but rather a cocoon. A safe cocoon in which I could sleep.

I began to explore the nature of the spiral. What is a spiral? Remember how, as a child, you used to have fun asking people to describe a spiral staircase without using their hands? It is such a three-dimensional concept that it is hard to describe it in flat, two-dimensional language. I used to think of psychological growth in that way, as a kind of spiral staircase. I noticed that people—myself included—seemed to return to the same old psychological problems and issues again and again, even though they had previously "resolved" them. It seemed that although they had been resolved at one level, they kept reappearing at new, perhaps higher, levels. I found this a satisfactory explanation at the time, and for that time it *was* satisfactory.

I realize now that it is in the nature of the Western mind to think in linear terms. In Eastern thought, everything revolves in circles, but in the West we always have to be going somewhere. Up or down, straight ahead or backward, it does not matter which, as long as there is a direction to it. The spiral of growth seems to have been our way of incorporating linear, forward movement with the Eastern concept of circularity.

These days, I no longer have such certainties about the issues of growth, progress, or evolution. I simply know that we must enter fully into whatever is our experience in the moment and see what that moment brings. However, I know that somewhere in my mind, the notion of the spiral of growth is still a guiding paradigm. I am, after all, a westerner, steeped in Western modes of thinking. Though I may have studied Eastern ways, I can never turn myself into what I am not. I have to accept that my mind has been shaped by notions of linearity and progress. At the same time, it is important to accept that linearity is only one way to construct reality. Once we fully accept that both concepts are equally valid, we can view the world in a new and more open way.

By acknowledging the relativity of all ways of thought, we can see a world in which linearity is simply a choice among other choices, a perception of reality that differs from other perceptions, a preference of one particular culture. We can then feel free to use our own culture's modes of thought, its metaphors and concepts, without being constricted by them.

I speak of these things so that you will remember that what we are speaking of here is a metaphor for experience, not a description of reality. Moreover, it is a metaphor for *my* experience, and for the experience of some other women I have interviewed, but it is not necessarily an experience you will have shared. I offer it to you, but I do not wish to impose it upon you. Treat it, if you will, as a myth, or a teaching story, which may hold some meaning you can harvest for your own life. Let me speak to you of the inward spiral and the cocoon, and see if there is anything in these images which may be useful to you on your own journey through menopause or in your own understanding of others who are making that journey.

The discovery of the cocoon was a surprising one. Once I envisioned the spiral with a cocoon at its center, everything began to change. A cocoon is, in a way, a place of rest, almost a place of death, for it is a place where some creatures go in order to die out of their previous form. Thus it is also a place of rebirth, a place from which the new form, in its own time, will emerge. As I read and talked to other women and explored my own process, I gradually began to discover that the whole experience of this time of life, for a woman, is like a death and rebirth. Ursula LeGuin said: "The woman ... must become pregnant with herself at last. She must bear herself, her third self, her old age, with travail and alone. Not many will help her with that birth."[1]

In the course of my research on this subject, I have asked many women about their experiences of this life stage. Those experiences are woven deeply into the fabric of this book. You will hear many voices as we progress through our contemplation of all the aspects of menopause. These women shared their thoughts and feelings, their hopes and fears and inspirations, and even their drawings. Some of them drew spirals, as I had done.

As I share with you their experiences and my own, I invite you now to explore with me the idea of menopause as a spiritual adventure, a journey, maybe even a transformation of the deepest kind.

1

WHAT IS MENOPAUSE?

What *is* menopause? Is it only that my monthly periods cease, my fertility ends, and my body begins to dry out and grow old?

Is menopause merely something that happens to my body? Or are there changes, also, in my thinking and my feeling, in my way of being in the world and in the meaning which my world holds for me? And if so, how do I deal with them and what lies at the end of it all?

These were the questions whirling in my mind as I entered this strange new phase of my life journey.

I thought about it a lot. I looked it up in books, for that was the way I had learned in my childhood. If you want to know something, look it up. Start with the dictionary.

My dictionary defined menopause simply as "the physiological cessation of menstruation." I discovered that the word had arrived in our language around 1872, and literally means "cessation of the menses," from the Greek words for "month" and "cease." The word was an import from France, where it was apparently coined, and where it had been used in medical literature early in the 1800s. It did not appear in an English dictionary until 1887.[1]

So was that it? No more blood—was that all? What was all my fuss about? Were all the strange new feelings, ideas, and dreams that erupted in me at this midpoint of my life a gen-

uine part of menopause, or were they the symptoms of neu-
rosis or worse?

I looked at my own family history. For my mother, yes, the
cessation of the menses defined it nicely. For her that had
been all there was to it, or so she said. I struggled with that
knowledge, wanting to be like her, like all those who "breeze
through" such happenings and seem to look askance at others
who cannot do likewise. Nevertheless, I began to speak my
own truth, despite some feelings of embarrassment at first.
As I did so, I started to hear the echoes in other women's
stories.

Much as I love my mother, I am not my mother. For me,
so much of life has been different, and my writing is a way
of honoring that. So, beginning with my own experience, and
rippling out into a sharing of the experiences of others, I have
studied menopause, and all that it is, above and beyond the
cessation of menses. In so doing, I have made for myself a
deeper, wider definition of that word.

For me, menopause has now come to mean much more than
simply the physical ending of menstruation. It has become a
special and very rich word—a word which denotes not merely
a biological process, but rather a whole stage in a woman's
life. It includes all that is happening within and around her.
I am not simply "having" my menopause, I am living it. Thus
all my living is a part of it, either actually or potentially.

In the way I shall use it in this book therefore, the word
menopause describes a holistic experience which encompas-
ses not only the dwindling away of the monthly bleed but all
the other phenomena which cluster around this very basic
fact of life, and all the subjective feelings which may accom-
pany it.

This experience may include hot flashes, strange new emotions, dreams, depression, elation, bodily changes, alterations
in thinking patterns, and much, much more. Or it may include
absolutely none of these. It is an experience which may last
for many years, which may begin long before the periods
actually cease at all and continue long after their ceasing, or
it may be over and done with in a matter of months, or hardly

even noticed. It is this wide variation which, for me, makes the whole subject so fascinating.

In the chapters which follow, when I speak of menopause, my emphasis will be not on the physical cessation of periods but on the time of life which surrounds and contains this phenomenon, a "change of life" rich with opportunities for self-awareness, understanding, and growth.

I did not always think of it this way.

* * *

A long time ago—I suppose it would have been about twenty years ago now—I chanced upon a pink-covered book in my local library. I do not know what drew me to that particular book on that particular day. But I remember that it was a book about menopause. It was written by a medical doctor and it spoke of revolution. Revolution in which no woman need ever again suffer the discomforts and indignities of menopause. Modern science, said the good doctor, had conquered menopause. Henceforth, women had the right to live to the end of their days in a new way, in which nothing was lost and much was gained.

I was in my early thirties then, with young children. My skin was as yet untouched by wrinkles; my hair was brown and glossy. Within me, estrogen surged each month. It felt so good to be me, so satisfying to be in this rich, juicy, female body. And here was this book, promising me that it would now be possible, with the new hormone replacement therapy, to stay that way to the end of my days. Nature might have had this cruel plot to start writing me out of her script in another fifteen years or so, but here was my opportunity to take charge of my own script, to rewrite it with myself remaining in the starring role.

Inspired, I wrote a glowing review of the pink book and submitted it for publication in a journal to which I regularly subscribed.

The editor was a retired doctor in her early sixties, a woman whose life and ideas I had long respected and admired. To my surprise, she greeted my offering with a total absence of enthusiasm.

"Menopause," she told me firmly, with a no-nonsense gleam in her sharp, blue eyes and a sterner-than-usual note in her deep doctor's voice, "is a *natural event* and should remain that way."

I was so taken aback that I withdrew my book review and retreated to think about the whole matter.

It was not long, however, before I had convinced myself that my friend the doctor was just an elderly reactionary and that my generation held the tools of liberation in its hands. I, too, would take hormones when the time came. After all, I reasoned, this was not unnatural. It was simply a replacement of something natural, like dentures or insulin, like contact lenses, or the brown rinse that I may one day choose to put through silvering hair. The matter was settled. My plans were firm and my future was—like everything else—under my control.

I smile today, remembering it. She is dead now, the stern-voiced doctor with her short, gray hair and her spectacles, and her "old-fashioned" ideas. She died, in reality, a decade ago, but for me she died as a guide and inspiration that day when she spoke to me from the other side of a chasm I had no intention of crossing. I judged her, dismissed her, reasoned her out of my plans for how life ought to be. My generation was going to do it differently. We were going to stay in control of our lives.

It is only now that I realize the importance of surrender.

* * *

One of the things which makes the study of menopause so confusing is the fact that it is but one factor in the overall process of growing older. Many things are likely to be happening in our outer lives at this time. Inwardly, too, both men and women are likely to experience changes in themselves as they reach their late forties and fifties, changes for which people of both sexes are often ill-prepared. As Carl Jung so eloquently said,

> Thoroughly unprepared we take the step into the afternoon of life; worse still, we take this step with the false assumption that our truths and ideals will serve us as hitherto. But we cannot live the afternoon of life according to the programme of life's morning.... How many of us older ones [are] really prepared for the second half of life, for old age, death and eternity? ... The afternoon of life must also have a significance of its own and cannot be merely a pitiful appendage to life's morning.[2]

Jung wrote these words in 1930. Even then, of course, there was nothing new about the idea of life as a sequence of stages. Remember how Shakespeare spoke so poignantly of our "exits and entrances" in the theatre of life? Bound, as we are, into our perceived relationship with linear time, we cannot but see life as a developmental sequence, a series of changes, through which we grow. Infancy, childhood, adolescence, adulthood, middle age, old age, death—each may be seen as a phase to be completed. A phase, that is, with special tasks to be done, particular challenges to be faced. A journey, with mileposts to be checked off. A lifetime-long board game to be played, at the end of which is an uncertain prize.

Millions of words have been spoken and written about these processes of change. Jung speaks of processes which occur in the human psyche as the individual passes the significant markers of mid-life and moves toward the gateway of old age. The markers are there to remind us of the constancy of change and the inevitability of that last big change—death.

Men and women may choose to ignore or deny the changes of aging. Deny them they often do. The middle-aged man buys a toupee in defiance of his balding head. The woman pays for a face-lift in defiance of her wrinkling skin. New partners may be sought; new ventures may be begun as a few extra dreams are desperately gleaned from between the last remaining stubble-stalks of the adult harvest.

For all our fierce denial of our aging, there is one change which cannot be denied completely, and that is the woman's physical experience of her menopause. Willy-nilly, the monthly process of ovulation will eventually stop, and, unless we take hormone supplements to continue it, so will the familiar phenomenon of menstruation. We cannot pretend that it is not happening.

Perhaps it is because of the undeniable nature of this change that most of the literature on menopause is so closely focused around the physiological, hormonal issues and so little is written about all the other changes which women, specifically, may experience as part of the whole process.

To alter the physical effects of the change needs deliberate medical intervention. Many women are, of course, ready to make that intervention, and thankful for it. Whether we choose to intervene or not—by the incorporation of replacement hormones into the body by pills, injections, implants, skin patches, and so on—there is no way that we can deny the fact of menopause, even to ourselves. If we do intervene, then the consciousness of our intervention, the very fact of undergoing the therapy, serves to remind us that the hormones which now circulate within us are no longer produced by our own bodies but are taken in from the outside. We are something new, the creation of twentieth-century medicine. We cannot pretend otherwise.

In our culture, the language of menopause nowadays is medical language. Rejecting the dusty remnants of folk wisdom that hint darkly at the horrors of "the change of life," we turn thankfully toward the bright, fluorescent light of medicine to make sense of the happenings within us. Even if we choose not to intervene in the hormonal processes, our very decision is more than likely informed by medical knowledge. We turn to medicine with all our questions.

Medicine, as always, obliges us with neat, scientific explanations, inviting us to use its clean, sterile words, its language of sign and symptom, cell and system, biology and biochemistry, diagnosis and prognosis.

So easy to fall in line. Yet such a trap. For if we are not very careful, language can lead us away from our experience. The map can be mistaken for the territory. Our thinking, feeling, experiencing life can become a catalog of symptom and solution, condition and cure, a two-dimensional living that can no longer deeply satisfy. A loss, perhaps, of soul. For the medicine of the West does not speak the language of the soul.

Language is so much more than a convenient way of communicating with others. It is a potent force which shapes the way we think. And in its turn, the way we think shapes our experience. The way we think and speak of menopause defines its meaning for us and defines the limits of what it may teach each of us in her own life. This is why, in the following chapters, I have deliberately chosen to speak of menopause not in the language of medicine but in the language of my own body and my own soul, and I invite you to do the same.

That is not to say that medicine has nothing to offer. It has much indeed. However, I believe that in order to live our lives fully we have to remind ourselves to go within as well as without, to seek for wisdom as well as for knowledge, and to learn to blend the two in order to answer our own deep questions.

There is much to learn of our bodies. Some is learning that comes simply from living in them. We could perhaps call that "body wisdom." Then there is the legacy of knowledge, passed on in each generation, and in each generation swollen by the contributions of a legion of diligent workers at the rock face, the scientists who labor continually to mine the knowledge-gold and add it to the pile we inherit.

Out of habit, the habit of our schooling in society, it may be that pile of received knowledge to which we first turn, rather than to our own inner wisdom. Do we seek out the wise old woman who lives in a cave under the hill, saying, "Please tell me about menopause, now that my time has come?" Or is it more likely to be a clean-looking medical graduate in a white coat who ushers us politely into his or her consulting-room and hears our first uncertain questions?

Any woman brought up in our modern Western culture, regardless of her formal schooling in the physical sciences, is likely to seek some level of "scientific" knowledge in seeking to learn about menopause. She may seek it from a friend or from a magazine article or from a radio or TV program. She may buy or borrow a book of some kind, whether it be a popular book or a medical or biological text. She may consult someone whose level of scientific knowledge she perceives to be higher than her own, such as a physician or other health professional.

She almost certainly believes that if she is fully to compre-

hend the changes taking place within her she needs a basic
understanding of the hormonal systems which govern the
menstrual cycle. The books and articles she reads and the
people she consults will usually oblige that belief. Most books
on menopause devote considerable space to exploring this
complex interplay of body chemicals, usually in the first chapter. In this book, I have deliberately avoided doing that. Not
that these facts are not important or worth knowing. On the
contrary, they are fascinating, and we should know them. But
I believe that they are masking something even more fascinating. I want to take us beyond hormones.

I must admit that when I first decided not to include a
chapter on hormones, I was not clear about my reasons. I love
knowledge and have always sought it greedily. I have university degrees, a whole wall of crowded bookshelves, and a
curiosity as insatiable as any two-year-old's. Yet, as I go
through menopause, I feel the stirring of something new and
different inside me that does not arise out of knowledge or
from the medically defined facts of my body, though it is
intimately connected with them. I do not know what this new
something is, and yet, to my dismay, it seems almost to want
to displace my knowledge at times, like a young usurper of
the throne.

The days when I feel the presence of this strange something
usually happen to be those days when my knowledge has
chosen to desert me unexpectedly, inexplicably, leaving me
floundering. Days when my mind goes blank and questions go
unanswered. Days when I blush and panic at my inability to
respond, wondering why my mental filing cabinet is suddenly
jammed shut, my inner computer "down" and silent.

At first, when I began to have such days, I struggled and
fought, trying vainly to get my knowledge systems up and
working again. It was only when I gave up the fight and settled
into a strange new inner silence that I began to feel little
stirrings of that new way of being that still has no name. And
because of my wish to honor and explore this new way of
being, I decided to approach the whole question of menopause
from a slightly different angle. This is the angle of surrender.

Surrender, that is, to a natural process, in order to learn its deepest lessons.

I had experienced childbirth that way. Now I wanted to experience menopause that way. So, eventually, do I hope to approach death. In fact, the more I think about it, the more I realize that it is the way in which I would like to approach every single moment of my life. To surrender into it. To live like that is to be fully alive in every moment, I believe.

That is not to say that I now believe hormone replacement therapy to be wrong. I think it has much to offer many women. The point about living one's life fully in every moment is that one is totally free to make choices. I could easily have chosen to take hormones and explore the process which resulted from *that*. That, also, would have been a form of surrender. The reason I did not is that for me the alternative was simply more exciting.

My decision not to write about hormones was, in a way, a symbolic one.

To commence a book on menopause with a treatise on hormones sets the tone of the book. It implies that menopause is primarily a physical condition and that the mental, psychological, emotional, and spiritual changes which may take place are in some way "side effects" of physiological, chemical changes in the body.

We are so conditioned to thinking this way that it rarely occurs to anyone to suggest, for example, that all this may be another way around. The physical may not be the most crucial element. By making it central, we imply that it *is* the most crucial, and somehow the other aspects of menopause get lost or ignored or at best "put up with," rather than examined and used for self-awareness and growth.

Just imagine that our theories were different. Suppose, for example, that there were subtle changes taking place in the psyche of a fifty-year-old woman which would lead, within a few years, to a decrease in her estrogen levels and cause her periods to stop. Think about it. Visualize a theory which said that certain thoughts and feelings, frequently experienced, might perhaps create impulses in the cerebral cortex of the brain which would affect the hypothalamus. This in its turn would create a signal in the pituitary gland, causing chemical messages to be sent to the ovaries and estrogen production to decline. Is this a totally implausible theory? What if, in fact, my periods were stopping because of my feelings of turbulence and change? What if my ovulation had ceased because of an order from my soul?

Please understand that I am not putting this forward as serious scientific theory, but rather as a way of jolting you out of your habitual ways of understanding your feelings and experiences. A way of making you look again at familiar things and see them in a new way. Seeing old things in a new way is one of the factors which helps us to grow.

As a rule, science says very little about causation. Scientists are careful people. They are very careful about making claims that something causes something else. It is usually sufficient to note that certain things frequently go together with certain other things. People may draw their own conclusions about what causes what. The trouble is, we human beings are very keen on the idea of causation. We are always asking questions with "why" in them. And even though our scientists are careful with their "because" answers, we often scoop up their findings and turn them into cause-and-effect answers for ourselves. Particularly about things which concern us intimately, like the workings of our bodies.

I am not suggesting that we doubt our scientific knowledge of physiology. We know an enormous amount about the workings of our bodies nowadays, including the workings of our reproductive systems, and that knowledge is immensely valuable. Knowledge almost always is. The trouble is that it can sometimes get in the way of wisdom, in the way of our ability to listen to our own inner experience and define our own answers, to create our own theories, to follow our own deepest inner guidance.

We in the modern Western world have come to rely very heavily on our knowledge in the last few hundred years. Ever since the early scientists began to put forward the notion of the world as a giant clockwork machine whose parts could be disassembled and understood, we have been entranced by the idea that one day we may perhaps understand *everything*. So we have studied, dissected, explored, experimented, and on and on, convinced that one day we would know the whole. Slowly, in the last few decades, we have begun to realize that we never can. Like the donkey with the carrot tied to the front of its nose, we can only travel down that path; we can never arrive. Not because the machine is too complicated, but because the world is not actually a machine at all. We have been following the wrong metaphor. The world is more like a living organism. Some say it is, in fact, a giant living organism. And like any other living organism, it is more than the sum of its component parts. Just as you are more than the sum of your body cells and their processes, so is our world more than the sum of its atoms and its natural "laws." There is, and always has been, something else above and beyond the accumulated knowledge and clockwork rules and the sum of the parts.

Perhaps it is my sense of that something else, whatever it is, which is trying to push its way up through the piles of knowledge in my mind, like a new shoot forcing its way up through the mulch of last year's fallen leaves.

Of one thing I am sure. And that is that my experience of menopause is more than the machinations of my hormones. It is longer and wider and much, much deeper than the happenings in my physical self. Yet it is intimately tied to them, and it is undeniably a female experience, for I am not simply speaking of the universal human experience of growing older.

What, then, is this experience of which I speak? What is menopause if I do not simply accept the biological facts as central and everything else as a side effect? In other words, what is menopause if we look at it holistically and yet maintain that it is something essentially female?

This book is an attempt to answer that question. In the course of the attempt, I shall be drawing on three sources of data. The first is my own personal experience of menopause as foreshadowed in the Introduction, when I spoke of the inward spiral and the cocoon of metamorphosis.

The second is the documented experience of all those other women who have made their experiences available to me, either informally as friends or as psychotherapy clients, or by taking part in my own research studies, or by writing and telling their stories for publication to the wider world.

Paradoxically, the third and most important is the experience of you, the reader, for it is only through your own life that my words can assume meaning. Like the liquid one adds to a cake mix, it is your contribution to the whole which brings it alive for you and gives it its substance and reality. For this reason, there will be exercises at the end of each chapter which invite you to explore your own unique set of thoughts and feelings, your own experience of menopause, whatever that may be.

In my own searching, I began with medicine. In fact, when I first began my reading I, too, accepted the conventional wisdom that menopause was a medical "condition," with "symptoms." I accepted that all the other things commonly associated with menopause were simply side effects of the physical, and thus, naturally, that the people who knew most about all this were the doctors.

However, the more deeply I read into the available literature, the wider my mind opened to other ways of understanding the whole phenomenon of menopause.

The first thing I discovered was that the way a woman experiences menopause is to a great extent defined by the culture in which she lives.

It is rather like laughter. The ability to laugh is universal amongst human beings yet the sense of humor varies greatly from one country to another. Likewise, the bare biological fact of menopause is common to all women but the way it is understood and experienced in each woman's consciousness is certainly very different, and some of the differences appear to be cultural.

Even the biological common denominator is only the fact that every woman's period stops eventually. The timing is different for everyone. In modern Western industrial societies, this usually happens somewhere around the age of fifty. It is uninfluenced by racial background, physical characteristics, or any other factor so far determined except cigarette smoking.[3] I discovered, however, that there are other societies in which studies have found whole groups of women reaching menopause in their thirties and forties.[4]

One researcher, investigating menopause among rural Mexican women on the Yucatan Peninsula, found that more than three-quarters of them had started their menopause before the age of forty-five. Furthermore, when asked about hot flashes, those sudden rushes of body heat which are so familiar to most menopausal women in our culture, the Mexican women not only did not report them, they had no term in their language to represent the phenomenon. For them, hot flashes apparently did not exist.[5] So much for biological universality.

If the biological facts themselves can differ between populations, how much more different must be the subjective experiences?

Anthropologists have suggested that one important factor in the way women view menopause concerns how it affects their feelings of value, or self-worth. There are societies, for example, where the postmenopausal woman is given access to information and opportunities previously denied her. One such example occurs in the Druze of the eastern Mediterranean region. Women in this society who have passed their menopause are initiated into the esoteric secrets of their religion, a privilege normally reserved for men, and thus attain special status in the spiritual life of the group.[6]

The well-known anthropologist Margaret Mead reported that in many of the societies she studied, postmenopausal women came to be treated as men by the rest of their group. No longer set apart by their reproductive function and its mysteries—and the taboo of menstrual blood—they were at last able to enjoy some of the same freedom that men had.[7]

There are other cultures, however, in which it is not an advantage to reach menopause. Many Muslim women in Mediterranean countries live with the knowledge that the end of their fertility may be the signal for their husbands to look for a second wife. One researcher reports that for many of the women he has studied, this creates anxiety of neurotic proportions.[8]

Interestingly enough, as this same researcher notes, the condition of "worthlessness" which menopause creates for women in some cultures, for example, in parts of black Africa, may actually be turned by them into a kind of advantage. He says, "An enemy would no more consider it worthwhile attacking her than trying to kill a worthless animal. Therefore, she need not fear the anger of ancestors, the malevolence of evil spirits, nor indeed infection by disease. She can undertake the most hazardous tasks with equanimity."[9]

For this woman, her menopause brings her a strange new immunity, even as it robs her of her former status as a person.

We must bear in mind, of course, that for most of history the majority of women did not live much beyond menopause anyway. Recent research involving the examination of Neanderthal skeletons lends weight to what we have always suspected: Modern women are the only female primates to live far beyond the end of their reproductive capacity.[10] Little wonder, then, that in many societies such few postmenopausal women as there were could simply be absorbed into the group life of the men or else given special ritual status. Or that they could, like the black African woman, become marginal "nonpeople" who could flit soundlessly between the structures of their group without being noticed or valued.

What of ourselves and our own times? Just as menopause may seem to vary greatly in its meaning and its implications from one culture to another, so are there variations between different groups of women within our own society.

Modern Western society is composed of so many diverse cultural and subcultural strands that we can expect to find a wide variation between individuals as well. In addition, we are a society which, in modern times, has come to place great emphasis on individual development and freedom, in contrast to many tribal societies. We are also a society whose female members have a reasonable expectation of living well beyond their menopause, and this, too, is a historical "first."

For all these reasons, it is difficult, if not impossible, to generalize about the meanings which our own peer group assigns to menopause. We can only speculate and ask.

It is thus with great caution that I offer in this book my own speculations and the answers to some of my asking.

I must admit that sometimes it feels strange to think of myself as part of a group that barely existed before. Like a new hybrid variety of being, I occasionally visualize myself as some odd, new creature, cut off from the comfort of precedent and tradition, forced to create my own folkways, my own meanings. This feels sad, lonely, and alienating.

Yet at other times, those self-same facts add up to something which is exciting and interesting, like exploration or pioneering. Perhaps it depends on what mood I am in at the time.

As I mentioned before, when I began researching the subject of menopause I saw it, as so many others seemed to, in a medical framework. Later I began to question this more and more deeply.

Of course we all know that menopause is not a disease. However, it is indexed in the World Health Organization's "International Classification of Diseases," and there is certainly no doubt that amongst certain sections of the medical fraternity it is defined not as a natural process, like being born or reaching puberty or dying, but as a "hormone deficiency condition" which may be corrected by the use of hormone replacement therapy.

Looking back to the history books, we find that menopause started to enter the medical domain in English society around the turn of the last century, and somewhat earlier in France. Before that, although it was accepted that this time of life could bring problems, the acknowledged expert on the subject was the traditional wise woman—the midwife. Why medicine began to take over that role is a larger and even more fascinating question, but one which I do not choose to diverge into at this point. It is connected to the suppression of the ancient Goddess religions and men's fear of female power, and we shall return to that topic in Chapter 7. Suffice to say here that medicine has taken a keen interest in menopause for quite some time now, just as it has in birth and all other aspects of female reproductive functioning.

In the 1960s there was an enormous surge of interest in the use of hormones to alleviate menopausal symptoms—not only the hot flashes which many women found unpleasant, but the disabling, and sometimes fatal, osteoporosis. This is a condition for which menopausal women are at a higher risk than the general population, according to the current conventional wisdom in medical circles, since estrogen is reputedly connected to bone density. In osteoporosis, bones lose density and become brittle.

Following the medical research and drug trials, a flurry of popular books appeared putting forward the notion that women were no longer doomed to what was often seen as a sort of premature "wearing out." It was one such book that I had chanced upon in the library. That book with the pink cover.

Now, years later, as I reached the threshold of menopause myself and began to think about it and to question and to read, I found some of these books, still in print. I read again about the danger of growing old before my time. Like this extract, written in 1971, by a (male) doctor. Carried away with enthusiasm for the wonders of the estrogen pill, he called it "one of the early steps in medicine's attempt to produce a wife who doesn't wear out. Furthermore, it will give women a tremendous psychological boost knowing they finally have something other than the artificial support of make-up to help them keep up with their husbands."[11]

How much I must have changed in the last twenty years. Far from offering me hope and relief, the revisited language of those books, so dated now, revealed itself to me as pompous, sexist, and insulting. I felt patronized, and very angry. This may perhaps have been the beginning of my decision *not* to take hormones. It was certainly the beginning of my determination to find what lay outside that way of thinking known as the "medical model."

Suddenly, I did not want doctors—particularly male ones—intruding into menopause, studying it, dissecting it, "fixing" it. I wanted to explore it secretly, just as in my childhood I had explored my girl's body, alone and in my own time. I wanted, too, to explore it with other women, in that same special sisterhood with which we began our puberty. "What did you feel?", "Was it like this for you?", "Me, too." I wanted to re-own it, as something essentially female and nonmedical. And so I went searching, without and within.

I began to write down my dreams. I began to spend time alone that was specially devoted to exploring the new and often jumbled feelings. Using pastels and huge sketchbooks, I started to draw the images of menopause.

One day, I found myself dancing the feelings, wordlessly turning my living room into an outer model of my life and dancing within it my fears of moving on, of growing old, of dying and taking final leave of my children.

Sound arose in me, sometimes tuneless and harsh, like a wild, despairing scream, sometimes soft and lilting, like a lullaby. In song and poem, in music and in words, I expressed what was happening in my life and slowly began to understand it. Deep in the safety of my cocoon, I was learning to come to terms with the changes in myself, in my thinking, my feelings, my way of being in the world.

As I spoke of my inner journey to other women, I discovered that I was not alone on the path. Several women told me that they had been able to arrange life in such a way that they were free to remain in their cocoons of self-discovery for weeks or months at a time. Fortunate in having the financial means to do so, they had temporarily withdrawn from the world of work in order to concentrate on the inner changes.

Others were banding together, forming groups in order to share their feelings and explorations. Over and over again, as I expressed my own thoughts and feelings, I found others like me.

In contrast, I found many who were struggling and afraid, many who were defensive, many who dismissed my words scornfully. I also found that, for the majority, the medical framework was the only one they had when they attempted to construct a meaning for menopause. I began to explore this issue with increasing interest.

I discovered that the so-called "medicalization of menopause" was a hotly debated issue, particularly among feminists. However, unlike the medical takeover of other natural processes, such as childbirth and death, this one was proceeding fairly slowly.

Although the "disease of menopause" has been created, it seems that we do not all believe in it—yet. In order for the medicalization process to be completed, there must be a total switch. In other words, women would need to move from total reliance on themselves and each other and a personal, nonmedical "support network" to a reliance on the medical system for defining and managing the "condition." So far, it seems, this has not happened, and medical opinions on menopause are formed only on the basis of women who report "symptoms" to their doctors—not, as yet, a majority.[12]

The meaning of menopause is still defined by women themselves, influenced though it may well be by the trickle-down from medical to popular journals and other mass media. I noticed, for example, that although they frequently saw menopause in medical terms, fewer than half of the women I have questioned have actually consulted their physicians about any menopausal issues. When you consider that virtually every pregnant woman goes automatically to a doctor and that death, by law, is something only a doctor can—and must— define, you can see that menopause has not yet been totally medicalized in the same way that birth and death have been.

The "biological revolution" promised by hormone replacement therapy must have tempted a lot of women into accepting the medical model unquestioningly in the 1970s. However, as time went on and carcinogenic side effects began to show up in the research statistics, enthusiasm for this new way of handling menopause began to be tempered with caution. Popular books now began to appear which took the opposite stance, encouraging women to be cautious about the hormone revolution. They suggested that one should consider the facts carefully, and that it may be preferable to let menopause proceed naturally, unless symptoms were so unpleasant or debilitating that some medical intervention seemed warranted.[13] Many of my generation have been confused about the facts, and still are.

The debate about hormones still rages. It has become more and more complex as more discoveries are made about the effects of hormones, in different combinations and dosages, on various organs of the body. Doctors are loudly debating the differential risks of such conditions as osteoporosis, thromboembolism, endometrial cancer, and cholecystitis. Medicine is still trying to get it right, still trying to perfect the "treatment." The race is on for the "perfect" therapy. There is big money to be made.

How are we supposed to choose? To make a fully informed decision on the subject is becoming increasingly difficult for the layperson, who is thus at risk of reliance on the information currently available in popular literature or on the personal bias of her own physician.

To make matters worse, studies have proved that the physicians themselves, far from being the unbiased scientists of our imaginations, are subject to an equally wide range of influences both in and out of the medical institutions and are every bit as shaped in their thinking by the cultural myths and folk models around them as are any of their patients.[14]

Even within medicine itself, preoccupied as it may seem to be with the heroic stance of "curing" menopause, there are a few who are pondering the question of individual meaning. At an international conference on menopause held in Belgium in 1981, one of the stated conclusions was that "the menopause is not an independent variable but a social construct, the meaning of which is created and sustained through processes of human communication," and that "it is important, if greater understanding of middle-age and the menopause is required, to study ... the ways in which women assign meaning to middle-age in general and to the menopause in particular."[15]

If the debate on hormone replacement has created a lot of soul-searching for some menopausal women, at least the majority have been free to decide their own course of action. About a quarter of the women I have questioned are or have been on some kind of hormone replacement therapy; however, most seem to be doing it very cautiously or only minimally, such as using topical estrogen cream. Some women have told me they are investigating various herbal alternatives. One woman reported taking an eight-month herbal class specifically so that she could experiment with estrogen herbs "so that I can stop taking artificial estrogen."

Another woman, a nurse, had been on hormones for six months because of fears of osteoporosis. Tests had shown her to have decreased bone mass. However, she stopped. Despite the benefits, she no longer felt right inside, and to her that was the most important thing. She said, "I felt heavy and not myself." So she is taking extra calcium instead. "I'm not happy about taking hormones until I'm 89! I'll take my chances with fractures," was her conclusion.

One woman described her process thus:

> While I am free of the side effects of menopause, I cannot honestly believe I am suffering. I do not take any medication as I am not convinced that the short-term gain is worth risking a long-term unnatural change. (The female body is so finely tuned it's hard to believe that Nature would let us down during or after menopause.) I have discussed the question with both a male and a female doctor. Interestingly, the male laid out all the facts and passed no judgment; the female (young) pushed hormone treatment. In the end, I trusted myself.

My questioning revealed many such individual decisions—decisions to trust an internal wisdom, to take chances rather than chemically alter the body's juices in an unknown way.

The women who are not quite so free to make their decisions about these matters are those who have had menopause thrust upon them by surgery. When a woman's ovaries are surgically removed, the physical effects of menopause begin to happen with alarming suddenness. In this situation, she has little choice but to start artificial hormones if she is not to be overwhelmed by the immediacy of the change. The problem is, as many women have found out, that medical science is, as yet, far from expert at duplicating the effects of naturally produced female hormones in the body. Therefore, a woman who has been finely attuned to the workings of her body now finds herself at the mercy of dosages and of the challenge of getting them right. Failure to do so can create a crisis wherein she no longer feels as though she is inhabiting the same body. She might even begin to wonder who she is. Not for her the slow descent into the center, the patient weaving of the cocoon. For her it is an outer hand, with a surgeon's scalpel in it, which has hurled her into chaos. To take up the challenge she perhaps needs more courage than all the rest of us. If you are one such, then I salute you.

If we decline to use the medical model to make sense of our experience, what can we use instead? After all, as I said before, the biological events of menopause are the only part of it which can easily be dissected out from the whole mishmash of issues about aging in both sexes. And certainly, as we can see with surgical menopause, there are such strong connections between our hormones and the way we are emotionally and psychologically that we cannot deny the importance of our endocrine systems in the whole thing. This is why it is so tempting to stay with the medical approach and with all the research that it has produced.

If removal of the ovaries can change us so drastically and so fast, then what are we? Are we, after all, merely a function of our own biochemistry? In a way, I suppose, you could say that we are, in the same way that you could do a chemical analysis of our fleshly bodies and discover that we are composed of 80 percent water. Yet, if we pay attention to our insides, somehow each of us is able to recognize the configuration of a familiar self in the subtle movements of our hormones. Artificial hormones, however carefully administered, may still create a feeling of not-self. "I felt heavy and not myself."

There is so much to learn, on so many levels. I feel as though we have only just begun.

Then there are the social aspects. For most of us, it is very likely that other significant changes will be taking place in our outer lives at the same time that the hormonal changes are happening on the inside. Children leaving home, parents becoming old or sick or dying, and so on. Inasmuch as menopause is a clear signal that we are entering the doorway of middle age, it tells us that now is the time to recall all we have learned in our lives about human development and aging. Now is the time when we have somehow to make sense of it, in real life rather than in theory. Now we begin to feel what it really means to be older, to join the older ones, to see our children move on, to touch death.

If we set aside the whole problem of what causes what, and simply look at menopause as a stage of life, like puberty, then all these other things become part of it. We are redefining ourselves. At this point in our lives, we have the opportunity to become intimately aware, more poignantly than ever before, of the relentless, universal imperatives of change. We are changing. Our bodies are changing and so are our psyches. Our environments are changing around us. We *are* change. It is scary, perhaps. But it is also one of our grandest challenges. Learning to surrender to the inexorable process of change, year by year, month by month, moment by moment. This can be our lesson.

So from now, for the rest of this book, when I speak of menopause I am speaking of the whole package and whatever it may contain. Whether it is your "empty nest" or your emerging wrinkles, your thinning hair or your feelings of gloom or elation, your thoughts of death, your hot flashes or your moments of pure zest, whatever it may be, it is part of what we are talking about.

Menopause can mean many different things to different people. It is a physical fact and a life stage. It may even be a frame of mind. It may have mental aspects, affecting the way we think, and emotional aspects, affecting the way we feel. It may also have deeply spiritual aspects, creating a total transformation in our deepest being, if it is consciously chosen by us as a vehicle for such transformational work.

Above all, it is important that each one of us should create her own personal definition of what menopause means for her rather than be bound by medical, cultural, or any other predetermined definitions from the outside, including mine. Trust your own experience. Go with it and see where it takes you. It can never be wrong.

In this chapter I have described some of my thoughts, feelings, and experiences concerning menopause. Now it is time for you to look within and begin to discover what menopause means in *your* life. Your ideas and feelings may be similar to mine or they may be very different. Whatever they are, they are totally valid and extremely important. I honor and respect them and I ask that you do likewise.

Experiment: What Does Menopause Mean to Me?

First, use your thinking mind.

You will need four sheets of paper and a pen or pencil.

Since menopause is, above all, a time of change, I am suggesting that you take careful note of exactly what changes are happening inside you right now. All of them. List them even if you do not believe that they are "connected" to menopause. Remember, when we talk of menopause in this context we are talking about an entire era of your life. So *everything* which is happening to you right now is relevant in some way.

Label the first page PHYSICAL CHANGES. On this page, list every single thing which is changing about you physically at this time.

The second page is headed MENTAL CHANGES. Have you noticed any mental changes lately? These may be changes in your patterns of thinking or the way you use your mind. They may be in the content of your thoughts or in the process of thinking them.

Write down any such changes you have noticed.

The third page is for EMOTIONAL CHANGES. This means changes in feelings, changes in moods, and so on. It may be changes in the ways you react to people or interact with them. These may be changes you have noticed in yourself or changes that others may claim to have noticed in you in recent times. (Write those down, too, even if you do not agree with what others have been saying.)

The fourth page is for SPIRITUAL CHANGES. This might mean changes in the way you see your life's purpose, changes in whatever it is that gives deeper meaning to your life, beyond the everyday tasks and problems. It might mean changes in your spiritual practice, in your beliefs or values, your religion, and so on, if you follow one. List here the changes which are happening to you on the deepest level, if indeed you have noticed any. If not, that is all right, too.

Take your time about listing these. You may want to put them aside for a while and come back to them later. Other thoughts may come to you at a later stage. If so, take time to add them to your list.

The second half of this exercise involves the intuitive part of you. To do it, you will *not* need your thinking mind. In fact if your mind feels very active now, because of your reading of this chapter, it may be better to leave this part of the exercise until later, when your thoughts are quieter.

Once again, you will need a sheet of paper, the bigger the better. And something to draw with. Colored pencils, pens, or crayons would be ideal, or even paint. I like pastels best.

On your sheet of paper, draw a large rectangle. Imagine that this is the cover of a book. Write the title somewhere on the cover. The book is called *A Woman's Experience of Menopause*. Now you are the graphic artist who has been commissioned to illustrate this book cover. Without using your thinking mind, simply illustrate the book cover.

Use whatever colors, designs, or pictures come into your head, without thinking about them. You do not need to be an actual artist, or have any drawing talent whatsoever. You can use abstract designs, patterns, symbols, stick figures—whatever you like. Let your head go and put down whatever spontaneously comes, without censoring it. Work at it until you feel an "Aha" feeling, or some emotion rise up within you, and you know that you have captured the essence of something. If nothing comes, you may wish to leave it for another day. Or just sit and contemplate that very sense of nothingness. Whatever comes, it will be right. Stay with it as far as it goes, whatever it is. There are no right or wrong ways to do this or any of the exercises in this book. There are no points to score, no marks to earn. There is only yourself to go into, more and more deeply, as we travel together.

You may like to leave your answers for some time before looking at them again. When you look at them, imagine you are someone else, someone who is seeking to know that person who wrote and drew the words and pictures on those pages. Let the words and drawings speak to you. Let your intuition play with them, as though they were a dream whose meaning will gently unfurl itself in your conscious mind. You do not need to work at it too hard. It will come of its own accord, as meaning always does if we relax and let it happen.

In the following chapters we shall examine all these aspects of menopause—the physical, mental, emotional, and spiritual changes—and how we can learn from them. They are the stuff of which our metamorphosis is made. They are the fibres of our cocoon.

2

WHO AM I? WHAT AM I MADE OF?

I believe that there are certain moments in our experiencing of our physical, female bodies that imprint themselves, like snapshots, in the memory. These experiences imprint so deeply that with each of them we feel ourselves irrevocably changed, as though we had passed through a doorway into a new place.

Perhaps this is because, for many of us, they are the moments which bring us back into deep connection with our ·bodies—events which are so physical and immediate that we have to allow them into our awareness of the moment. We cannot sleep through them.

Take a moment to recall the uniquely female, physical feelings which may have been strong and meaningful for you. The first sexual experience, maybe. Or pregnancy and birth. If you have borne children, call to mind once more the quickening, the first flutter of the new life inside you, like a bird moving in the hand. If you have given birth by natural methods, you may recall the unbelievable energy of the birthing womb. If you have suckled a child, you will remember, I am sure, the tingling joy of milk letting down, the sweet soreness of nipples. Recall the various feelings and sensations of the menstrual cycle. The fullness and wetness of ovulation, the swollen tenderness of premenstrual tissues, the dragging ache of a heavy period, the "whoosh" of a sudden clot of blood leaving the vagina.

Some time, when you have the opportunity, ask another woman about those certain moments in her life. Ask her about the first time she saw her own menstrual blood. Now *that* is a moment. Different for each of us, yet for most of us it was one of those snapshot moments. Was—or is. Is, because those moments are a part of the eternal present. We carry them onward. They are part of who we are.

I was surprised at how brown it was. I expected that it would be red. Mothers don't tell you everyday details like that. Well, maybe some do, but mine did not. Just the mechanics of it, and how to affix one of those old-fashioned, cumbersome pads to an elastic belt. She gave me two of the pads, and a belt, wrapped in white tissue paper, all in readiness.

I remember the excitement of that tissue-wrapped packet that waited for a full two years in my top dressing-table drawer. Waiting, waiting, waiting for that special moment to arrive. In a way it was a private waiting, an inner waiting which I did not fully comprehend, any more than I comprehended the other changes that were happening to me. The new turbulence in my thoughts and emotions, the strange new flashes of feeling, and strong, unfamiliar stirrings. There was a certain ritual, spiritual quality about that private waiting. The tissue-wrapped package seemed like the icon of a strange, new religion of which I had, as yet, no knowledge. It looked so awesome and different, sitting there in my drawer, amongst the familiar objects of my life, the brush and comb and hair ribbons of my known, physical world. I took it out and handled it sometimes, gingerly, with a kind of scared reverence. It seemed to fill the drawer with its strangeness, its withheld meaning, through all those interminable months of waiting.

The public waiting, though, that was different altogether. "Have you got it yet?" my friends would inquire eagerly each day. "Anything *happened?*" That made the waiting longer, having to say "No" each school morning for such a long time. Menstruation, in that outer, public face of high school, was spiritual in a very different way. It was the spirituality of initiation, of blood sisterhood, of the inner circle that I longed to join, and its litany was pure tradition. The girls sitting huddled by the radiator with their groans and cramps, the mystique of, "I can't go swimming today." In those pretampon days, the ones with their periods sat on the grassy hill above the swimming pool, in the sun, while the others swam. Their names were listed in a book and checked for regularity to prevent cheating. Swimming lessons were the highlight of my week, and yet how I longed to sit on the hill. I wanted my name in that book; my signature, in blood, recorded into history.

Blood must never actually be visible, however. There was always a dread of "accidents." That night of the gymnastics display, I can see it again now. One of the senior girls, our best gymnast, dressed all in white, running up to perform a flawless vault, to the applause of several hundred assembled schoolchildren and their parents and families. As she flipped upside down, a frisson ran through the assembly hall. I can feel it now and see, still clearly, the little blood-red stain that the whole school saw with horror and pity. At that moment it felt to me as though her life had been ruined, her star status gone for good. "Oh poor thing, how awful!" was on everyone's lips.

What a strange taboo we live under. Yet it was not until I began researching menopause that I realized there was a taboo there at all, so thoroughly had I absorbed it myself.

Paula Weideger, in her book *Menstruation and Menopause*,[1] explains that in many primitive societies, menstrual blood was thought to possess special powers, and the menstruating woman was often feared by men. Elaborate taboo systems were constructed to protect other people from this powerful magic. In some groups, women were secluded in special huts during their bleeding, out of sight of the rest of the tribe. There were strict rules about what the woman could do or not do during her period.

We notice, with a sophisticated amusement, the many traces of these taboos which remain today. We may see the more primitive ones on our travels. In Bali, Indonesia, for instance, there are notices posted at temple doorways re-

questing that women not enter the temples during their periods. Women in many parts of the world believe that they
cannot cook certain dishes at these times. A woman in Ma-
laysia told me that if, while she was menstruating, she made
the special sweetmeat of fermented sweet rice wrapped in
banana leaves, it would emerge blood red and be unfit to eat.
Religions have "purification" ceremonies, ritual baths, and
so on. Many of us remember the old wives' tales of our grand-
mothers. My own grandmother told me I should never wash
my hair during my period.

We smile at these relics of the past. Yet how many of us
realize how totally we have, in fact, internalized the menstrual taboo? What is your own reaction to the sudden sight
of another woman's menstrual blood? How carefully do you
hide all signs of your own from the public eye? We take responsibility upon ourselves for keeping the whole process of
monthly bleeding discreetly out of sight. The artist Judy Chicago noted in her autobiography *Through the Flower* that she
and a group of friends, discussing menstruation one night,
suddenly realized that there were never any images of it in
art. It was as though the phenomenon did not exist, even
though it is the universal experience of half the human
population.[2]

We may not think often of these things, of taboos and memories, of rites of passage and the significance of our blood. But
when we do think about them, those snapshot memories stand
out. Menarche, the first bleeding, is a rite of passage with a
mood and feeling all its own, different for each of us and yet
in some ways similar, for when we hear each other's stories
there is usually a deep recognition. The events may differ but
there is something universal nonetheless, and we feel it when
we share.

Rites of passage, in the sense that the anthropologist Van
Gennep coined the term back in 1906,[3] are both outward and
inward events. Outwardly, they mark society's recognition of
a change of status; inwardly they mark the progress of the
soul. Physical events such as the ones we have mentioned may
be rites of passage for many women in an inward sense, even
though they may not be outwardly acknowledged by society.

This lack of acknowledgment is particularly noticeable in our modern Western society, which, as the late Joseph Campbell lamented, has lost many such opportunities for social ritual.[4]

That feeling of passing through a doorway into a new place is the inward experience of an important rite of passage. If we can be consciously aware of such passages, even if only in private, our lives, I believe, will take on a richer meaning.

As women we are no strangers to change, for we are constantly in flux. We are, above all, cyclic creatures. Esther Harding, the Jungian analyst, writes of the psychic energy in women which waxes and wanes with the moon: "These energy changes affect her, not only in her physical and sexual life, but in her psychic life as well. Life in her ebbs and flows, so that she is dependent on her inner rhythm."[5] Yet we are taught to "overcome" our cyclic natures—as though it were possible! How did this come about? Well, for one thing, women in Victorian times were seen as weak, fragile creatures with their own strange "female" problems that made them incapable of doing many of the things which men could do. Feminists, over two centuries, have worked to dispel this notion, with considerable success. There are very few human enterprises now, at least in Western societies, where women have not staked a claim alongside men. We have successful women in every walk of life and a large percentage of the work force is female. This is wonderful progress, but we have paid a price.

The work force is based on machinery, and machinery is based on straight-line efficiency—on even, consistent output, unchanging from day to day. Women run on a monthly cycle. Not only their bodies change, but their feelings, moods, energies, and abilities change. There is a constantly moving rhythm, not only of hormones but also of perceptions, emotions, even dreams. In order to fit into a "male-ordered" world and prove that they are "as good as men," women have had to override their natural rhythms by willpower. They have had to ignore and suppress their natural, rhythmic ways of being as best they can. They have usually succeeded, but they have sacrificed something in order to succeed. The menstrual cycle has been "coped with" rather than enjoyed. PMS has been something to dread and seek to remedy rather than an opportunity for inner work and spiritual growth. Monthly periods are a nuisance at best and painful or embarrassing at worst. For the sake of the Gross National Product, and to prove the point that we can do anything men can do, whether it is scaling Everest, walking in space, or being a prime minister, we have learned to subdue our biology. Since we are, by nature, so governed by our biology, this means we have had to split away from ourselves.

Our splitting away has been quite an unconscious experience for us. We are often not aware that we have an option. The fight to control the cyclic process has become part of what most women accept as normal. For many women of my generation, being able to ignore menopause has been a triumph rather than a missed opportunity.

The women I interviewed about menopause were asked, first of all, what they felt about their years of menstruation. For many of them, it was simply a hassle. They had struggled with pain, discomfort, embarrassment, ruination of social plans, worry over contraception, premenstrual tension, and stress. Above all, the struggle had been to "get through" it each month and return to "normal" as quickly as possible.

For the women of this type, who were in the majority, the saving grace was that it enabled them to have children, or at least to have the option of childbearing. One woman, who had completed her family, expressed it thus: "Once I had the two children I wanted . . . it was an awful waste to have to keep going through this rigamarole each month." If she believes in the reality of regular, consistent, ordered world, based on the machine paradigm, a woman's cyclic changes are a constant challenge. As another woman expressed it: "I want to get on with life and two weeks of each month being physiologically slowed down I hate." For these women, cyclicity is something which must be constantly battled with or "put up with" in order to conform to the greater rhythms of the outside world.

The second type of woman, very much in the minority, was one who, despite the disadvantages, welcomed and celebrated her rhythms. She seemed to be a woman not only at home in her biology but revelling in it. Like this woman, for example, who says that she felt

> somewhat different at different stages, but generally I have had feelings of contentment. Somehow I have felt reassured at the regularity of my cycle. Despite periods of discomfort, and so on, I realize that I have always kept track of my cycle. I felt it was an important part of being a woman.

Or this one, who, although she suffered a lot of PMS symptoms which, she said, made life very stressful, added, "However, I also liked the rhythms, especially when it was exactly at full moon or new moon." This woman also mentioned the positive, sexual feelings at ovulation, and another described "almost a 'born again' feeling—almost euphoric—like I love everyone and everything and all is well and good." She would not, this woman emphatically stated, change places with a man.

For these women, cyclicity was accepted as the nature of their being. Females, after all, came into existence long before machines were invented. Our cycle is prior to all man-made cycles and is an intrinsic part of who we are. We repress it at our peril.

Penelope Shuttle and Peter Redgrove, in their 1978 book *The Wise Wound*, claim that it is this forced splitting of ourselves and suppression of our rhythmic, changing nature which is actually the *cause* of menstrual pain and PMS.[6]

Perhaps that sounds farfetched. But let us think about it for a moment. Let us think about the question of definition. How you define something will profoundly affect the way you experience it. We create our own reality from moment to moment by the way we define things.

Those who have experienced natural childbirth will remember that one of the key features was the way in which the feelings were defined. Those bodily sensations, particularly the birth contractions, were overwhelmingly strong sensations. The study and practice of natural childbirth methods did not lessen the strength of the contractions. What it did was redefine them. Rather than experiencing the body as a body in pain, a body gripped by alien forces, and therefore contracting against the sensations, one learned to experience it as a body *hard at work*. A body working harder, probably, than it had ever worked in its life; this is labor in a very true sense. And working in a way that was healthy and natural, a way that the female body usually knows instinctively how to follow, if we do not hinder the flow of it. So, instead of shrinking away from the sensation, you breathed into it. You went with it, like a surfer riding a wave. The sensations of labor, when experienced this way, are no less strong, but totally different. You cannot call it pain, yet you cannot *not* call it pain. It is qualitatively different. It hurts, yet it does not hurt.

It is not necessary to have given birth to understand this principle. Here is an experiment in redefinition.

Experiment: Playing with Redefinition

You will need a small towel, a dishcloth, or some other piece of fabric which can withstand rough treatment. Hold this in your two hands. Imagine that it is dripping wet. (If you want to be even more realistic, you can wet it, but then you will have to figure out how to avoid getting the book wet!)

Grasp the material very firmly, and begin to wring it out. Your task is to wring every single drop of water from that fabric in one single squeeze. Focus your attention totally on the purpose and the goal. Try to use your hands alone, rather than your arms and shoulders. Squeeze as hard as you can.

As you reach the point where the very last drop is coming out, maintain the action as hard as you can. Hold it just there. Now, still maintaining full pressure, switch your awareness to the physical sensation in your hands. Look at your hands. Observe their color, their appearance. Are they stretched in places, red, swollen? Become exquisitely aware now of *just* the sensation in your hands. Imagine that you had been simply sitting quietly and your hands had begun to ache like this for no apparent reason, all by themselves. Imagine that some strange disease of the muscles had caused them to grip spasmodically in this fashion, a disease over which you had no control. Feel the sensation now as pure *pain*. Let yourself be aware of how much pain there is in your hands right now.

Can you feel how your perception of the sensation changes as you switch your focus from the task of squeezing out the cloth to the pure experiencing of pain? Did it switch from "hard work" to "pain"? Now switch it back. Finally, let go and relax.

You may want to do the experiment again without reading it at the same time so that you can concentrate on the sensations. Play with it. Switch it back and forth. See how interchangeable the concepts of pain and hard work are.

This is how natural childbirth works. What may have been pain becomes simply hard work.

Shuttle and Redgrove explain that by defining our periods, our PMS, and all the rest as "symptoms," as conditions to be coped with or stifled, we have unwittingly created pain and stress. If we had learned, right from the beginning, to breathe into them, live them fully, and explore them for what they could teach us, our experience might have been altogether different.

If we can apply this technique to menopause also, then our experience of this stage of life and its "symptoms" may be completely different from what we had expected. How would we experience a "hot flash" if we had defined it differently? Let us play with that idea for a moment.

Do you remember what they said to you when you were a teenager, struggling with new feelings, new sensations, acne perhaps, or emotional storms? Did they ever say, "Don't worry, your body is just undergoing a whole lot of changes right now"? These may have been your own words to someone, a teenage daughter perhaps, a niece, a pupil, a young friend.

This is equally true of menopause. The fact that we are older and wiser and have probably practiced downplaying our menstrual lives for forty years does not mean that we shall not experience as much turbulence at the cessation of fertility as we did at its commencement. For some of us, there may be more. After forty years' addiction to our own estrogen, we may well be suffering withdrawal symptoms. We are undergoing another radical change, a time when the actual cells of our body will change in certain ways, just as the cells of the caterpillar inside the cocoon will change, quietly and in darkness.

Imagine yourself inside the cocoon. Imagine that it would be possible to *feel* the changes happening. Like a crucible, that cocoon of change needs heat in order to create the metamorphosis within. Suppose that the next time you had a hot flash you could pause and go within, and redefine that spreading, burning heat as the heat of change? The next time it happens, try it. Feel the fire that is rearranging your cells, the creative fire of your metamorphosis into the woman you will eventually become, a woman whose menstrual blood will have changed, alchemically, into wisdom. Feel your heat in this new way. Go with it. Let it take you over. Surrender to it. Let yourself change. It may take many blasts of heat before the change is complete, but that is alright. Let it be so.

You may like to employ this same technique with any other physical discomforts you are experiencing at this time. Aching joints, itching skin, insomnia—any of these common menopausal "symptoms" may be redefined as metamorphic processes. We cannot know what happens to the caterpillar while it is inside the cocoon, nor what feelings it may experience there, but our imagination can play creatively with the idea that it feels all sorts of strange and wonderful sensations as it slowly undergoes its transformation. Like the caterpillar, we can feel them, too.

For some people reading these words, the idea of going deeply into physical experience in this way may be a new one. You the reader may be feeling some resistance or some puzzlement.

Let us pause for a moment, therefore, and consider how we may benefit from focusing on our bodily sensations to this degree.

Rather than attempting an intellectual explanation of my point of view, I am going to suggest another experiment. This time, there will be no pain, nor even hard work. It should, instead, be pleasant and relaxing. You will need at least ten uninterrupted minutes to do this experiment properly.

Experiment: Sensory Awareness Exercise

First, guarantee yourself ten minutes of uninterrupted peace and find a quiet, comfortable place to sit.

Let your body relax.

Take note of how you feel—physically, mentally, emotionally and so forth, *right at this moment.*

Record this overall feeling in your memory.

Now, begin listening to the sounds which are all around you. As you listen carefully, there will be many sounds—perhaps quite a few you had not noticed before. Listen as you would to music—open, receptive, accepting. Focus all your awareness on this symphony of subtle sound. You may want to close your eyes for a few minutes and leave the book in order to focus totally on the sounds. Do that now . . .

. . . Now your eyes are open again, returning to the page. Let your eyes begin to take in information, just as your ears have been doing. Let them leave the page and begin to wander around the room or wherever you are, exploring, taking in everything. Explore slowly, carefully: every color, texture, shape—lines, edges, patterns. Look at things as though you have never seen them before. Do it without defining them, without thinking about them. Just see them, each object, each surface, each shape, totally new, like a baby seeing the world for the first time. Explore. Leave the book now and go on your visual journey . . .

. . . Now begin to turn your awareness to the inner world. Begin to notice your body. How it feels inside. The pressure of the chair or whatever your body is resting upon, the temperature of the air, the odor of the surroundings. Do not label, simply experience.

Be aware of your hands, your feet. . . . Explore all the physical sensations that are coming in from all parts of your body; the taste in your mouth, the rhythm of your breathing. Are you hungry? Thirsty? Hurting? Are there parts that ache or itch or tingle? Explore. . . . Become fully open, fully aware of every inch, every cell, fully receptive to every feeling. Leave the book and take some more time with your body . . .

...Finally, try for a few moments to do all these things together. Maybe two of them at first, then all three. Be fully open to the sounds, to the sights, to the sensations, all at once. Leave the book to do this. Ears, eyes, body...

...Now relax. And take stock once more. What is your overall feeling now? Does it differ from the way it was at the beginning of the exercise?

Most people, after this exercise, report feeling a sense of greater aliveness and deeper awareness. It is as though we spend much of our waking days half-asleep, and at times like this we realize how different it feels to be wide awake. For many, this realization, in itself, is sufficient justification for trying to stay more closely in touch with the body.

The human brain is receiving signals from the outside world and from within the body at a rate of literally millions per second. In order to make sense of this barrage of incoming data, we have learned to be selective in what we choose to perceive and to "tune out" the rest. This is an adaptive pattern, essential for our evolutionary survival as a species. We have needed—and still need—this ability.

Unfortunately, we have learned this selectivity rather too well. We know how to ensure that we will perceive only what we want to perceive. That is how, as women, we have been able to suppress the awareness of those "inconvenient" rhythms and fit ourselves into the male-ordered world of steady office machinery. And this is how we can, if we wish, "get through" these potentially turbulent years of menopause. Taking hormone pills, maybe, or simply "toughing it out," pretending that nothing is happening, waiting for it all to be over so that "normal life" can resume.

Of course not everyone will necessarily experience turbulence. As we saw in Chapter 1, women's experiences of menopause are extremely variable. Each of us is a unique organism. There are women—my mother was one—who apparently experience no menopausal "symptoms" whatsoever; no hot flashes, nothing. One day the period no longer arrives and that is all there is to it. There were some women like that who took part in my research. I remember one of them describing herself as "one of the lucky ones." There were many, however, who were not so "lucky," many who were struggling with hot flashes, night sweats, insomnia, fuzzy-headed feelings, strange bouts of weepiness, and inner turmoil of one kind or another.

The point is, if we wish to experience full aliveness we must each be who we are. If we are one of those symptom-free "lucky ones," and menopause presents no challenge to us, then that is just fine. Our challenges obviously lie in other places, perhaps in our careers, or in other life experiences. Challenge can present itself in ten thousand different ways. But if we are not so "lucky," if menopause does seem to thrust itself into our lives as a challenge—physically, mentally, and in all the other ways in which changes may manifest—then we need to acknowledge it. We need to honor it rather than repress it. We need to ride it all the way to the shore. To do otherwise is to risk sacrificing our aliveness and to miss a potential opportunity for growth.

If, as women, we choose to live in full awareness of every moment and every revolution of our cyclic, female lives, we have an opportunity to experience a particular kind of aliveness that is ours alone: "Coming to terms with the rhythm of women's lives means coming to terms with life itself, accepting the imperatives of the body rather than the imperatives of an artificial, man-made, perhaps transcendentally beautiful civilization."[7]

This kind of aliveness, the kind which comes from entering fully into one's own experience and going wherever it leads, is what Richard Moss has termed "radical aliveness." It entails the full embrace of everything rather than the selectivity of judgment. It therefore demands that we go as willingly into our pain and uncertainty as we do into our joy.

> The pain and uncertainty of life is not wrong. It is as right as the joy and wonder of life. The only thing we can do is knock upon all the doors. This is radical aliveness. We begin to face the little death of yielding ourselves more fully into life's immediacy. We can knock upon the door of our own experience and we can be sure that we will be answered.[8]

So if menopause brings you no challenge, there is no need to invent one. However, if it does bring one, as it has to me, then I invite you to take it up. Follow your own inner voice, for it is your best guide. We must be who we are. Refusing to let ourselves feel what we feel, trying to fit ourselves into some preconceived idea of who or what we should be, we do ourselves an injustice. Refusing to go willingly into the cocoon, if it beckons us, we lose a precious chance to be reborn.

3

WHO AM I? WHAT DO I THINK?

As I sit here at my desk, recalling the history of my life as a menstruating woman, it occurs to me that I am using my mind to take a body journey.

As you sit with your pen and paper, recording all the changes that have come with menopause, you, too, are using your mind, that remarkable piece of human software. Together, we are making body journeys which are really mind journeys.

With our minds, we have visited scenes from the past, the preoccupations of the present, and visions for the future. We have used our minds and their incredible powers of visualization and conceptualization to ponder upon and redefine physical experience.

Using our minds, we have thought about the meaning of menopause to women across the globe and begun to explore the personal meaning which our own menopause has for us.

Now we can watch ourselves perform the greatest trick of all, the trick of which only humans seem to be capable. We can use our minds to examine our minds; exploring in thought the very process of thought itself; exploring the possibility that even here, in the world of pure thought, there may be some subtle, menopausal change.

Descartes, that famous French philosopher, said, "I think, therefore I am." In his view, it is thinking that defines us as human beings. It was that very skill, developed through millenia of evolution, which set us apart from the rest of the animal kingdom. Not only did it set us apart, but in the minds of most people, at least in the Western world, it set us "above" and supposedly gave us the right to sit on the throne of that kingdom and boss all the other animals around. Since we can think, that argument went, we are obviously smarter than all the other species with whom we share the earth, and thus we are in charge.

Certainly, we appear to have more highly developed thinking powers than most other species, and certainly our domination of the world seems now to have become absolute. Humankind is victorious. However, if pollution, overpopulation, global warming, and deforestation—all the consequences of our human thinking powers, whether directly or indirectly—bring our species to extinction, that absolute domination will have been hollow. And if we weep for the species now extinct, for the forests destroyed and the fishless rivers, we must know that *Homo sapiens* has not been a wise and responsible ruler but rather a foolish and ignorant one. We must also begin to know, in these thinking minds of ours, that smart thinking does not make us superior. It merely makes us rash and arrogant. Knowledge is not the same thing as wisdom.

With our knowledge, we have tried to rule the world, and with our knowledge we have all but wrecked the world, bringing it to a state where, before long, only the rocks will remain, silent witnesses to our collective folly.

Our only hope is to search for deeper wisdom. Wisdom that lies beneath the crust of knowledge our science and technology have created.

Our thinking has brought us science, and science has brought us technology. Science and technology in our century have become overwhelmingly powerful. They have brought us mind-created objects unguessed-at by our ancestors, and a host of wonders and inventions. Unfortunately, they have also brought us a host of previously unimagined problems. We keep believing that more thinking, more science, can solve the problems. Yet perhaps it is not more thinking but some other process which will unlock the answers to those global problems. Perhaps it is humility we need, and the willingness to listen, in peace and patience, for the quiet voices of wisdom to make themselves heard.

Perhaps we should start listening to ourselves. Fritz Perls, the iconoclastic therapist whose ideas became so popular in the sixties, used to say, "Lose your mind and come to your senses."[1] His message was that our overconcentration on thinking has made us forget how to feel. He told us that we had forgotten how to listen to our bodies, honor our sensations, tune in to our inner voices, and hear the messages from the unconscious parts of ourselves. It was his attempt to show people how overemphasis on thinking can serve to stifle those voices and messages in the pursuit of some outer goal or other, and make us tense, sick, or neurotic in the process.

In the same way, in the nineties, there are those who are calling out to us all to tune in to the inner voices of the planet itself, to listen to nature, to learn from the other species who are part of the planetary family, to rediscover the wisdom of those who have always lived close to the earth and respected its ways, such as the traditional peoples of North America and other lands.

Thomas Berry, in his magnificent and inspiring collection of essays, *The Dream of the Earth*, invites us into this new listening:

> In relation to the earth, we have been autistic for centuries. Only now have we begun to listen with some attention and with a willingness to respond to the earth's demands that we cease our industrial assault, that we abandon our inner rage against the conditions of our earthly existence, that we renew our human participation in the grand liturgy of the universe.[2]

There is an important place for thinking in our armory of skills. If they had not been able to think—and think very clearly and efficiently—these men whose words I have quoted would never have been able to put their words forward to inspire us.

We must be careful not to dismiss the importance of our thought processes altogether, not to throw out the baby of mind with the bathwater of excess thought.

Likewise, if we had not, as a species, evolved our thinking—and consequently our science—to the level which it has reached today, we would probably never have arrived at the point where we could share our knowledge, our information, and our concern with others on a worldwide basis. One could argue that had we not developed this facility of thought, we would never have been able to see our world as a whole, for the horizons of our thinking may have been limited to the boundaries of our villages and towns, our concerns limited to survival and the defense of our little pieces of territory. Certainly, we would never have been able to photograph our planet from outer space and see it hanging there in the dark sky, in all its blue and gold beauty, veiled in mist, a vision to unify all humankind. Life would have been very different. Worse, perhaps, or better. Who knows? The fact is, we have become a thinking race, a race which values thinking so highly that we have defined ourselves in terms of it. "I think," said Descartes, "therefore I am." Perhaps the corollary would be: "If I cannot think, then maybe I do not exist."

So what are we to think about thinking? And what does it all have to do with menopause?

In my early work with some menopausal women in therapy, I noticed that they reported a certain kind of mental state that was new to them and often somewhat alarming. It was as though their normal thinking patterns were disrupted for hours or even days at a time. One woman described this with a very strong image. She said it felt as though her head were packed with cotton, so that all thought was muffled and clarity was gone. She called it "cotton-head."

I knew immediately what she meant, for I had experienced that state of mind at certain times myself. Those were the times when I would find myself stopping my car in front of a green light or forgetting the name of someone I knew well. I had observed that it was a phenomenon which only seemed to occur on premenstrual days. It appeared to be part of the whole PMS package—the fluid retention, irritability, tendency to be clumsy—all of that well-known syndrome which so many of us have encountered on a regular basis during our menstrual lives. I had even developed the habit of noticing, at the beginning of the day, whether or not I had that cotton-head feeling, and, if I had, I tried to avoid driving my car on that day. This seemed like a sensible safety measure, for I knew my driving was less safe at those times. Such routines are fairly simple to maintain when one is menstruating regularly, for PMS is a predictable occurrence and one can plan around it. But menopause is a different kettle of fish.

When my own menopause began, I discovered how it feels to have, not hours, but endless days of cotton-head. Days that could not be planned for. A thick, pervasive cloud immobilized my mind and sent me into a panic.

Around the time that I started noticing the apparent sudden increase in these cotton-headed days, I was involved in some research with families of patients suffering from Alzheimer's disease. I began to fear that I, too, had the disease, for surely there must be something seriously wrong with a mind that showed such obvious signs of deterioration in thinking quality.

I agonized. I fought it. I thrashed against the fog, screaming my protest, willing my mind to think crisply, clearly, as of old. Like someone trapped, I beat against the walls of my prison, only to fall exhausted at the day's end.

Who was I, after all, if I could not think? "I think, therefore I am." Who was I if I could not function? Who was this person lost in the fog? The interior of my mind looked different now, unfamiliar. I was a stranger inside my own head. I fought it long and hard.

I did not win the fight. But deep in the darkness a door began to open, as doors so often do when we stop struggling with our despair. This is how surrender works. It was the door to a totally new place, a place I had always wanted to find, but had never succeeded in finding, precisely because of that very mind I had prized so highly. My mind, my thinking, had kept me from surrendering, from passing through a door that was now, at last, opening to me. I began to explore, fearfully, with some wistful backward glances at the safety of the old, familiar places.

My new discoveries had two main features. The first had to do with cerebral hemispheres and mental functions. In other words, it concerned an organ very crucial to our ability to think—that strangely shaped, bone-encased, hardware whose gray-and-white mass of living matter we call the human brain.

The human brain differs from the brains of our closest mammalian relatives in a quantitative way. That is to say, it has a denser network of neuronal connections in its outer layer, the cerebral cortex. This cortex is apparently the latest section of the brain to evolve. As you look at the brains of simpler and simpler animals, you see less and less of this layer, though the inner structures are similar. It would seem, then, that as evolution proceeded, the "newer models" retained all the basic features of the older one, developing and specializing certain functions. We humans have evolved thanks to this thickened and deeply convoluted cerebral cortex, which gives us the ability to move from simple perception to a process of highly sophisticated and complex thought.

Our brains, as most people know, are divided into two hemispheres. These two hemispheres have a tendency to operate in somewhat different ways. The left, which controls the right side of the body, usually operates in a linear, rational way, rather like a computer. It is also the side predominantly involved with speech. The right, which governs the left side of the body, functions more holistically. It has little language ability but excels at anything to do with space and time, recognition of patterns, and creativity. It seems to be able to process many inputs simultaneously and to arrange them into a pattern, whereas the left hemisphere lines them up and deals with them sequentially.[3]

In the days of Descartes, the property of "reason" was valued very highly. So it was, in fact, not simply the function of thinking in general which defined our humanity and allegedly made us so special, but specifically that left-hemisphere type of thinking, the linear, rational, logical kind which proceeds from step to step in an orderly sequence. Although most of humankind's best thinking is done by people using both sides of their brains in a very integrated way, nonetheless it has frequently been reason which has received the credit. All through recent history we see evidence that the left hemisphere's specialty of linear, sequential thought has been highly prized and encouraged in our culture, at the expense of the equally essential right hemisphere's holism.

Our artists, with their right-hemisphere skills, have always been with us, in every epoch and culture, interpreting, portraying life in color, line, and form, in dance, music, and mime, in stone and bronze, or in simple scratchings on the face of a rock. Oh yes, we have valued them, but in a different way. So often, their contributions have been seen as peripheral rather than central to the main, grim business of survival and growth. Their work has entertainment value, but we rarely acknowledge the deep contributions of their vision to our unconscious life of myth and meaning.

This preference for rational thinking and the achievements of the intellect is conveyed to us through our parents and teachers, and naturally, to please them, we respond by learning to value these aspects more highly in ourselves.

If you doubt the truth of this process, look carefully at any school curriculum and see which subjects are deemed most "important." A child cannot help but be affected by this value system.

It appears to me that the heavier the emphasis is on the importance of logical, linear thinking, the more noticeable— and perhaps the more paralyzing—is the effect of the "cottonhead syndrome" on the individual. This is pure speculation, of course. I know, however, from my own experience, that the fogging over of logical, sequential thought and clear, rational speech is more devastating for me than the fogging over of right-brain functions like spatial arrangement and imaging. Presumably this is because my image of myself, created from the raw material of my childhood experiences, is the image of an intelligent, articulate person who excels at logical argument. These were the qualities that were admired and encouraged by my parents and others important to me in my

formative years, and therefore my self-image was built upon
an ideal of myself as someone possessing those qualities in
good measure. With the coming of menopause, more and more
holes appeared in this self-image.

First of all, it seems that the very ratio itself, the degree of
emphasis given to each cerebral hemisphere, is changing. I
am being drawn more and more toward activities favoring
the right hemisphere. It is as though an ancient balance within
me is being restored. Nowadays, when there is a spare moment, I no longer want to spend it thinking or writing. Instead,
I want to dance or paint. Even in my reveries, my moments
of lazy daydreaming, there used to be a train of thought, a
shuttle that carried the thread of ideas and gently wove my
tapestry of mind. Now I have learned to go down into the
vortex, where a thousand different voices sing, a thousand
different, chaotic visions swirl, and to do this with increasingly less fear. Slowly, steadily, I am learning to loosen the
reins of control, which had even extended into my formless
world of thought; I am learning to surrender.

As I mentioned in Chapter 1, Carl Jung made a study of the
second stage of life. He believed that there is a process of
development, of gradual becoming, which continues throughout the life cycle of the human individual. One factor in this
process of "individuation" is the particular mode in which
each personality interacts with his or her environment. Jung
noticed that there seem to be four main ways of doing this
and called them the "four functions:" sensation, thinking,
feeling, and intuition.[4]

Sensation is concrete perception through our senses. Event
X happens and we can see it, hear it, touch it, and so forth.
By thinking, we can conceptualize about event X. We can
figure out why it happened, who caused it to happen, and so
on. Feeling tells us whether we like it or not. It lets us know
where we stand regarding event X—whether we are delighted
by it or disgusted. Intuition provides a context for event X.
We may have known it would happen or we may guess that
it will happen again. We may intuit a connection between
event X and other events and not exactly know why.

All of us utilize these four functions, but each of us tends to favor certain ones habitually. This tendency is reinforced in early life. Parents who place heavy emphasis on intuition, for example, will reinforce the use of the intuitive function in their children, whereas thinkers will encourage thinking. As Jung saw it, one of the tasks of development is reclaiming the less-used functions as we proceed toward maturity.

If, as Jung believed, the process of individuation continues through the life span, it would not be surprising to find that at midlife there is an awareness of one's patterns changing. Naturally, they have been changing steadily since the day of our conception. However, at midlife, the focus is now shifting from the "doing" activities of the outer world to the "being" activities of the inner world. Therefore we are becoming more acutely aware of what is going on within us, physically, mentally, emotionally, and spiritually.

On the mental plane, we can now observe inner changes. The changing emphasis between the two "halves" of the brain, the reclaiming of the hitherto-neglected "functions" of which Jung spoke—these are balances which are being redressed. But if we do not understand what is happening to us, the process can be scary. We derive such comfort from knowing who we are. After all, it has taken us half a lifetime to establish that identity, that strong image of ourselves which we carry forever in our minds.

From the time that we first saw our toes waving at the other end of the crib and began to discover that we were individuals, through one billion interactions with others that defined us as *us*, we have been building this person that we think we are. There were all the books we searched through, seeking for descriptions of ourselves, all the magazine quizzes we eagerly filled out and the tests we sat through in an effort to determine our type, our personality, our style. There was the constant comparing of ourselves with others, both the real others in our lives and the fantasy, larger-than-life others of stage and screen. We have categorized ourselves in a thousand different ways. We have labeled and labeled, sorted and filed. We have constructed an identity. And by now we have become addicted to the comfortable feeling of knowing what it is. The knowledge of who we are has become our security blanket.

Menopause, which unglues the solid structures of our self-image, opens us to new possibilities. We can either fight to retain the old or we can open and embrace the new. This book invites you into that space and that embrace.

Patterns of thought, ways of processing the world as it comes into us, these are our most beloved of structures. They are the fixtures of our inner reality, the foundations of our self-image. When these structures begin to crumble and fall, there may be panic. After so many years of processing information in a certain way, the challenge of change in the mind can feel like catastrophe. I thought I had Alzheimer's disease, but it was simply the cotton-head syndrome of menopause and it brought with it the disintegration of one aspect of my self-image. What a gift that has proven to be, after all. My thinking, rational left hemisphere was finally ceding its place as boss in my mental kingdom; my thinking function was moving over to let other functions have a turn; and my self-image was asking to be reassessed. To me, all this has been a true gift, even though at the beginning it was hard to recognize as such.

How many of you have experienced this? I would make a guess that at least half of the women reading this book will have felt some significant mental changes that have come with this time of life. Look back at your answers at the end of Chapter 1 and see what you wrote under "mental changes." These changes may have been problematical to you, or they may not, depending on how important mental matters are to you, or to what extent you have defined yourself as a "thinking" type.

Out of all the women who have shared their menopausal experiences with me, there have been at least twenty percent who specifically described that feeling I have called cotton-head. They each found their own words for it. Several have called it "fuzzy-headedness" and others have labeled it "fuzzy thinking" or "fuzzy brain." Some named it "confusion," "disorientation," or "muddle." One labeled it "decreased sharpness of thinking." Some women say that they have difficulty in concentration and many report an impairment in memory. There have been others who named what I thought could

have been the effects of this syndrome rather than a description of the syndrome itself. For instance they have spoken of
greater difficulties in decision-making, an increased tendency
to procrastinate, and an inability to study. However, there
have been those who report less procrastination and *improved*
ability to study.

I notice that many women speak of a loosening of controls
over their thought processes. They find themselves saying surprising and unpredictable things. Some react with shock and
fear to this and try to grasp the controls more tightly, whereas
others find it amusing. I remember one who stated her obvious
delight in a new-found tendency to think and say "outrageous" things.

At first I was confused by the apparent contradictions. Why
would some people be experiencing a decrease in, for example,
their ability to study and concentrate, while others were experiencing an increase? Then I began to see that the essential
factor was change. The outcome of the change was less significant than the fact of change itself. Menopause, it seems,
has the potential to change our habitual patterns of thought.
It can change the shape of the boxes into which we have put
ourselves—and allowed others to put us—over the years. In
fact, it can blast us out of those boxes altogether. How we
respond to this new freedom, how we react to the feeling of
being out in the open air, standing by the remains of a pile
of firewood that once was a safe, secure box—that is what
makes the difference in our answers to the questions.

In some cases it may be that the splintering of the old self-
image is an instantly liberating experience. For other people,
there may be a longer period of clinging to the old. I suspect
that for the majority of us, change is usually frightening at
first, but as times goes on, the possibilities of the new become
attractive and exciting. The differences in answers may stem
from the fundamental differences between people and how
eagerly they welcome change, or it may simply reflect how far
the change process has proceeded in each individual life, and
whether or not its potential has been—or is being—explored.

This, then, was the first of my discoveries, the uncovering
of the changes in mental functioning and the freeing potential

which is inherent in such changes. After all, if I am no longer fixed in my ways of processing information, which dictate my ways of interacting with the world, then I am no longer bound by my old self-image, and thus there are possibilities for a new "me."

The second discovery went far beyond the idea of a new "me." It showed me a doorway beyond which there *was* no "me."

In one of the most famous metaphors ever created, Plato, the renowned philosopher of ancient Greece, spoke of a cave in which people were imprisoned. All they knew of life was the play of light and shadow on the wall of the cave. That was their reality and that, for them, was the whole of reality. All events in the outside world could only be seen by them as flickering reflections on the cave wall. They could never gaze directly upon those outside happenings and see them as they truly were.

This metaphor, the product of one man's mind well over two thousand years ago, is one of the great metaphors of all time. It is, in fact, a way of describing an idea of even greater antiquity. That idea may be found to this day at the center, the mystical heart, of all the great religions and belief systems of the world.

The idea is this. The reality that we humans think we perceive is not, in fact, reality. It is *our concept* of reality. It is reality as seen reflected on the inner walls of our minds. Reality, the true reality of the universe, is, by definition, totally beyond the ability of our minds to grasp. It is simply not possible for something as small, limited, and finite as the human mind to comprehend the great, unimaginable, and infinite vastness of the true reality of things. To attempt to comprehend something too vast for the mind is as stupid and futile as trying to lift oneself up by one's own bootstraps.

For one thing, in order to be able to process reality with these limited, finite minds of ours, we have to cut it up into manageable sections. It is similar to the way in which medical students, in learning to understand the human body, have to divide it up into categories, into pieces. They study subjects such as anatomy and physiology. Anatomy subdivides the body—hands, arms, heads, and so on—to examine the bones, muscles, and other connective tissues of which these parts are constructed. Physiology divides the body into "systems"—the digestive system, the circulatory system, and so on—and examines how they work. Despite all this carving up, the human being remains a whole entity. While Joe, the patient, is being carved up in the minds of the doctors into pieces and functions—Joe's circulation, Joe's small intestine, Joe's big toe— Joe remains Joe nonetheless. The reality of Joe is Joe, in his wholeness.

The basic, ungraspable fact is that all of reality is, in truth, as seamlessly joined as all the parts of Joe. What we habitually perceive as "all" is, in fact, one.

In order to grasp it with these little minds of ours, we have no choice but to cut it up in pieces, as the students mentally divide Joe. But it is not, in fact, a collection of discrete pieces. The entire universe is actually one seamless totality, as Joe is.

It is the direct realization of this seamlessness, this unity of all creation, which we call "enlightenment" or "grace" when, on some rare and beautiful occasion, an individual glimpses it and is forever changed by the experience. For the brief duration of that glimpse, reality is directly perceived, rather than being filtered through the dense screen of mind. In those moments, there is no subject and object, no observer and observed, no "that out there" and "me in here," no separation between self and other. All is one, and all boundaries are dissolved.

When Christ spoke of making "the inner as the outer and the outer as the inner and the above as the below" so that the Kingdom of Heaven might be entered, it was surely this of which he spoke.[5]

Likewise, during Buddha's great awakening under the *bodhi* tree, there was at last the understanding of the oneness of all things, and the illusory nature of the human concept of reality.

The Hindu scriptures, the oldest of all, have this truth as their very foundation. The disciplines which grew from them, such as Advaita Vedanta and the various forms of yoga, all aim at assisting the individual to pierce the veil of illusion and know the ultimate reality. In other words, they aid the individual in striving for the direct perception of reality, rather than the limited, partialized versions of it constantly produced by the mind.

So pervasive was this idea that Aldous Huxley dubbed it "the perennial philosophy" and gave examples of its existence somewhere at the heart of all the world's great religions.[6] In the everyday versions of those religions, lived by the vast majority of religious adherents, these ideas are often concealed from view. Being a Christian, a Jew, a Buddhist, a Muslim, a Hindu, and so on, is no guarantee of discovering the deeper truths. An atheist or agnostic may just as likely stumble upon them, and many do, I am sure. Many of the most spiritual people I have known have belonged to no organized religious group.

Most of us are so locked in to our concrete, partialized thinking, so trapped in the inner caves of our minds, that we cannot comprehend any other possibilities. We mouth the words and yet we miss the meanings. The teachings that we need are not esoteric teachings, hidden from sight; they are in the stuff of our daily lives, our everyday experience, yet we miss them, miss the opportunities for our own transformation.

It reminds me of the Sufi teaching stories, many of which are well-known at a popular level. They are stories whose words are written plainly for all to see. The deeper layers of meaning lie concealed, in broad daylight, in those very stories, yet we cannot see them until our eyes are opened in a new way. As one of the world's leading Sufis remarked, "The secret of Sufism is that it has no secret at all."[7] Likewise, the secret of experiencing reality is no secret at all, and yet so often it seems to us hidden and unattainable.

The urge to transcend mind and to gain that direct experience of reality is what powers the spiritual searchings of the second half of life, whether we realize it or not. From this, we can recognize the exciting possibilities presented to us by our menopausal changes in thinking.

If we find that our old concepts of ourselves are being demolished by the changes of the menopausal years, we have two choices. We can either build new concepts—new boxes out of the broken lumber of the old—or we can learn to be free instead. We have the option of constructing new identities. These will be new definitions of ourselves that make sense to us—new, updated images to carry around in our minds and live up to, and to refer back to in times of doubt. Alternatively, we can simply do without such reference points altogether. To do without them is to live in freedom.

To live in freedom means that we no longer operate out of a set idea of who we are. We are free to respond to every situation in whatever way seems appropriate to that situation, without reference to any image in our minds that has to be upheld.

Remember the woman who was surprised to find herself being "outrageous" nowadays? We could hypothesize that before menopause she had always been at pains to follow the guidelines of her self-image. She did not, as a rule, allow herself to do or say anything which overstepped those guidelines. Her responses to people and situations were usually predictable to herself, and probably to others, at least to those others who knew her well. Menopause, and the changing of her mental maps—the loosening of her need to stay on course—resulted in the tendency to stray into unfamiliar ways, and consequently she found herself being "outrageous" at times. It could happen that one day she will have ceased to notice how she is being. The sense of outrageousness will then have left her. She will simply "be." Still in possession of all her mental abilities, she will no longer be bound by any set ways of responding to anything. She will have opened the door to a higher freedom.

To respond in freedom means that we are not limited to the knowledge that we have stored in our minds. Instead of speaking from our minds and simply sharing knowledge, we can speak from our hearts. The words that come freely flowing from our hearts will be spoken from a place of wisdom rather than a store of knowledge. Though they may carry information, they embody wisdom, a deep knowing that goes far beyond the limited knowing of the mind.

When we interact with another out of a concept of who we think we are and, of course, who we think the other is, we lock ourselves out of this deep wisdom place. The interaction is limited, like the dialogue between two actors in a play, to the script dictated by the mental images we hold.

We do not only perceive the world through our mental concepts: we act out of them also. Not only do we carry around fixed ideas of who we are, we also carry fixed ideas of who others are. We stereotype, generalize, judge, and label. We become puppeteers, manipulating the papier-mâché representatives we have created to play the part of our "others," and to do our bidding. We can no longer see the other as he or she truly is. True reality is ungraspable and unpredictable; the true other is ultimately unknowable. It feels safer to stay inside and play with puppets. Barricaded into the tiny room of the mind, we can see the world only through the little windows of our fortress. Desperately seeking to control, we shout our orders through the slits in our mind-fortress walls, begging the world to be as we want it to be—safe, predictable, controllable.

How fortunate we are if, at menopause, our minds begin to let us down. We have an opportunity to start doing it all differently, to risk freedom, to surrender to unknowing.

So what began as cotton-head can be the beginning of a new and splendid challenge. These mental changes we are experiencing may offer an opportunity to abandon outworn concepts of who we are and to embrace a new freedom. These changes in our old modes of functioning present to us the possibility of becoming far less dependent on our minds than we have been before. In releasing that old dependence upon the mind, we may come to realize the severe limitations of the mind itself. Seeing the mind as limited can enable us, for the first time, to soar beyond it. This may be one of the most important opportunities we have ever had. It is the opportunity for spiritual transformation.

When we can reach beyond the limits of our thinking minds and begin to find our own wisdom, we become, in a sense, listening posts for the deeper wisdom of the earth as well. We are beginning, at last, to play our part in the great healing.

* * *

You may wish to spend some time pondering these thoughts about thought and how they apply to you.

Does your mind seem to become fuzzy at times, and filled with cotton? Are you experiencing changes in the way your mind works these days? Do you forget things you used to remember?

Perhaps you are an artist, a musician, a dreamer, someone for whom shape and imagery, poetry and form are more meaningful than words and concepts. If so, has menopause begun to bring changes to this style of being, and how does it feel?

Above all, who do you believe that you are? What are the definitions that describe your identity, to yourself and to others? Are they beginning to change?

The following is a powerful exercise. It looks simple, but it does have the power to change your whole way of being, if you choose to surrender to it.

Exercise: "Who Am I?"

The Indian sage Ramana Maharshi, who died in the 1950s, used to instruct his followers to ask themselves one simple question. The question was "Who Am I?"

They were not to ask it once, but many, many times. There is, in fact, no limit to the number of times one may ask it and the number of answers one can give in reply.

Try it. Ask yourself the question, and listen quietly to your own answer.

Let your mind rest gently on the answer. Ask it again. Answer it again. Listen to your second answer. Keep on asking it.

You may want to write down your answers, or simply to give them to yourself in words or thoughts and listen to them. Do not dwell for long on them, just listen to them, acknowledge them, and let them go.

When you slow down, or think you have come to the end of all the answers, keep asking the question. You will find that you can go on answering. As long as the question is asked, you can go on answering it.

If you run out of time, put the exercise aside and resume it later.

If, at any stage, you feel that you have come to the definitive answer, then simply listen to that answer and then continue. This is not the end of the process. Whatever feelings or emotions come up, let them emerge and be fully felt. There may be learning in this. Then move on. Resume your relentless questioning of yourself.

The same question, over and over. "Who Am I?" Keep answering, listening to your answers, and asking the question again. And again, and again.

It may take you many hours, days, weeks, or months before something begins to happen, but eventually something probably will.

You will feel a change, a shift. Just let that shift happen. Do not be hung up on results. Simply do the exercise and watch what happens. Whatever happens is all right. This is truly using your mind to liberate you from that very mind which shackles you. Seems crazy?

Try it.

4

WHO AM I? WHAT DO I FEEL?

Although the last chapter dealt with thinking processes rather than feelings or emotions, you will probably have found that the exercise at the end of it—the "Who Am I?" exercise—did not involve only thinking but brought with it considerable amounts of feeling as well.

Feeling and thinking frequently go hand in hand. The network of nerve cells which makes up the cerebral cortex, that outermost layer of the brain, is richly connected with deeper, internal brain structures, and it is within these deeper structures that the emotional centers of the brain are located. It is here that we feel pleasure, pain, rage, fear, and so forth.

Messages travel both ways along these busy communication lines. Thoughts can induce feelings and feelings can induce further thoughts. Thought and feeling dance together, sometimes urging each other on and on toward exhaustion. Can you remember dancing such a dance?

Perhaps it was the dance of worry. This a favorite with many of us, particularly those of us who are or have been mothers. Have you danced this dance? Remember that time you woke up, in the early hours of the morning, and realized that your teenager was not yet home? That was the thought which began it, the first step in the dance. Then the feeling came. Anxiety washed across you in a wave. You began to see pictures of automobile accidents in your mind (thoughts). The anxiety deepened and became dread (more feelings). You imagined the police car in the driveway (thought), and the dread came to the edge of panic (feeling), and so on.

Not all of us do the worry dance, but to some the steps may be familiar. I can dance it to the point of tears and exhaustion, if I allow it, particularly when the thoughts concern my children or when it is late at night and I am tired.

The only way to stop the worry dance is to separate thought and feeling from each other and ask feeling to move alone, without thought to lend its energy to the dance. Thus allowing my body to experience the feeling, I can break the cycle. Pure feeling, uninspired by further thought, dances itself to a quiet stop, if you can simply watch it with full awareness.

It is more difficult for thought to stand alone. Easy though it may be in arid, academic matters, or the pragmatic issues on our office desks, in the closer regions of our personal lives it is hard to have thoughts which do not also involve a component of feeling. Neither can we completely overrule feeling with thought, for feeling has its way of bubbling up through the thought layer like spring water, defying our attempts to dam it.

In the short term, however, we can have the illusion of success. There may have been many times in your life when you imagined you had successfully used new thoughts to smother some feeling state, either deliberately or in the general onward flow of events.

The feelings from a morning altercation with a family member, for example, are soon lost in the bustle of a day at the office. The disappointment of an empty mailbox is forgotten in absorption with the TV newscast. A crying child can be distracted with a toy. Thus, our purposeful attempts to suppress painful emotions by "thinking about something else" can appear to work. It really depends how deep and important the feelings are. If they are transitory feelings, reactions to the situations of the moment, they are contained in the moment and may also be obedient to the thought of the moment. Nevertheless, there is a danger of which we should be aware.

Even in the most fleeting feeling, there may be the potential for a residue to be left behind. Even a brief feeling, when suppressed, may trickle unnoticed into an underground storage tank. Over time, the tank fills, and one day, to everyone's astonishment, it suddenly bursts. Many marriages have been drowned by the sudden eruption of these underground tanks of feeling, imperceptibly filled over many years by the tiny trickles of unexpressed emotion.

We should therefore cultivate the habit of being totally aware of every feeling. Naturally, it may not always be appropriate to express it, but we should allow ourselves to feel it in its fullness rather than attempt to dam it up with a rationalizing thought and an injunction such as, "I shouldn't feel that way," or the popular, "I am just being irrational." Feelings, by definition, *are* irrational. This does not make them any the less valid, or important, than thoughts. As pointed out in the previous chapter, we have, as a society, set an arbitrarily high value on rationality. This has resulted in a certain lack of balance in many individuals and in the societies of which they form a part.

I am aware that I have been using the terms "feeling" and "emotion" somewhat loosely, and without defining them. Although dictionaries often give them as synonyms, in psychology there is a distinct difference between a feeling and an emotion. It is a difference which is quantitative more than qualitative. An emotion is a feeling which is accompanied by measurable, visible bodily reactions, such as crying, laughing, sweating, trembling, and so on. Any feeling may, in fact, produce some degree of bodily change, such as a tensing of muscles, but this might be so slight as to escape the notice of an observer or even of the person who is feeling it. Many of us are adept at remaining unaware of these little increments of tension. That is, until they compound into a headache or other painful symptom.

This is another reason why it behooves us to remain aware of our feelings and allow them to flow naturally through us rather than suppressing them. If we do not, the result may be physical illness.

As we have just seen, the place where feelings and emotions originate is in the deep structures of the brain. Down among these structures, seated on top of the hypothalamus, and intimately connected with it, is the pituitary gland, the so-called "master gland" of the body, which regulates the hormones, including those hormones which orchestrate the reproductive cycle. As women, we all know that our emotionality and the nature and intensity of our feelings vary according to our menstrual rhythms. There is obviously a deep connection between the hormonal activity of the pituitary gland and the feelings and emotions generated in the various centers in and near the hypothalamus.

At menopause, when the reproductive cycle is shutting down and great hormonal changes are happening in the body, it often seems that emotions become labile. It is almost as though the ability to repress and control is somehow lost. A new incontinence appears in our tear ducts. We weep where formerly we would have merely winced. Pleasure may turn to pain in minutes, or the reverse. The feelings flow unbidden, unchecked, uncheckable. The sphincter of thought cannot close on the stream of feeling.

So at this time in our lives it is quite usual to find feeling and thought whirling off into new dances, unchaperoned by the stern eye of rationality. And when this happens, all of our history begins to unfurl. All the unfinished business of the past comes up for reconsideration. We may revisit old pains long forgotten, old conflicts long-buried, old longings unfulfilled. This is the emotional business of menopause. This is the great task of this time of our lives and we must get on with it.

Does that sound daunting? For some of us, there is a weariness which descends from time to time, a deep fatigue which no amount of rest or vitamins can dispel. It comes upon us unexpectedly and may last for hours or days, turning everything we have to do into an effort. Even if our excitement and our motivation remain unchanged—and they, too, may desert us for whole chunks of time—there just is not the energy to carry out the tasks we have set ourselves. As if it were not enough simply to suffer from the cotton-head syndrome, we have the weariness as well. The weariness and the sudden, despairing feeling that nothing really matters anymore. It is an emptiness, an ennui. A gloomy place in which to find oneself.

Not every woman finds herself here, but many do. Some for just a brief while and some for longer. Some may be here and not recognize it, for it may be overshadowed by something larger, the death of a parent, for example. For some, I suspect that the work of the psyche proceeds by itself, below the threshold of awareness. However, I speak for myself and for the many who have spoken to me of these feelings of emptiness, weariness, and gloom.

It seems we have a confluence of three factors. There is the constant call to reexamine ourselves, our lives, and all that we have stood for previously, all that we have taken for granted up till now. There is the deadly cotton-head feeling, which turns our problem-solving into a muddled mental chaos, and finally there is the weariness that makes us wish we could drop it all and simply go to sleep.

Each of these three factors by itself may be devastating enough, but when all three converge, as they frequently do at this stage of our lives, the result can be a disabling depression.

So, you may be saying, here is this woman speaking of huge tasks, huge, new tasks of self-discovery. How can I do that when I can barely be bothered reading a magazine?

Do it we must. Whether we do it quickly or slowly, willingly or reluctantly, there is a task to be done. If we are to make the most of this opportunity for emotional and spiritual growth, then sometime around now we probably have to start cleaning out the cellar, even though we never felt less like cleaning a cellar in our lives.

We could decide not to clean the cellar. There may not be much in there, anyway. But for some of us, the junk in the cellar has become embarrassingly present. In our intimate relationships, in our interactions with others, and in the emotions these interactions bring up in us the junk is beginning to make its presence more strongly known. The things which upset us upset us more, and other things upset us which never used to do so. Adolescence revisited.

For me it has felt at times as though the junk from the cellar is beginning to erupt up the stairs, all by itself, rattling and bumping up the stairs, embarrassingly messy, dusty, and old. And it is coming to rest in the living room. Clouds of yesterday's dust in the living room of today.

Like it or not, if these emotional changes are happening to us, then there is nothing for it but to tackle the question of old junk. Old emotional junk. A lifetime's junk, coming up from the storage places in our psyches and sitting around in our lives. We start tripping over it. It begs to be wondered about, made sense of, and dealt with once and for all. It is a task which may occupy us for quite some time. Anything from a few weeks to several years.

Of course it is not the first time in our lives that we have been faced with the task of reviewing who we are at a feeling level. To some extent, the creation of ourselves as separate individuals, unique beings, has been proceeding steadily since the day we were born. There were certain stages in our lives, however, certain key points along the way, when the question of identity was the most important question in our lives, whether we remember it or not.

There was that time, somewhere between ages two and three, when we first realized our power and our separate will. We discovered "No." Discovering "No" went to our heads and for a while we overdosed on rebellion, just to be sure it was true that we were really free to decide, free to be different. When we finally became convinced of this, we relaxed and went back to learning about the world. By now, however, the idea of our selfhood was firmly implanted.

Then there was that time around seven when we discovered that the horizons of the family were not the horizons of the ocean. They were simply the edges of our own boats. So we began to make excursions out over the edges and away from the side, on to other boats. We began to be shaped by our peer groups and by the wider world that lay beyond.

By the beginning of adulthood, we had done much learning and experimentation. We had adapted to the demands of our particular situation, the idiosyncrasies of our family, and the requirements of our social group and culture. Our limitations and our genetic inheritance had determined some of the parameters. Some feelings and expressions were acceptable and some were not. However, we had also learned that there are many ways of being, many modes of feeling and expressing, many methods of living our lives and relating to others. Now it was time to start deciding who we really were and how we were going to be. It was time to go out into the world and stay there, and to stay in the world one must find a suitable set of clothes to wear in public. One must adopt a permanent identity. This key point seemed like a major one—and indeed it was.

As adolescents, on the threshold of adulthood, we had tried on various identities, modeling ourselves on the images presented to us by the world outside, copying others from our own personal world or the world of our popular culture. We had experimented. We strove to create The Look, The Image, from images on TV, in magazines, from the fads of the day, and from the people around us. We tried on this costume and that, self-consciously parading them in front of parents and peers, adapting, modifying, discarding, changing. A bit of this and a bit of that. Eventually, an identity of our own was formed. It was a blend of who we deeply were and who we wanted to be, a mixture of inheritance, experience, and intent. It gradually formed itself, as the feelings and tendencies of the real self underneath came up to stretch and shape the fabric of the costumes we had created to adorn the outside. Now, as we moved into adulthood, this was who we were and how the world came to know us.

These key periods in our lives—in childhood, adolescence, and early adulthood—were crucial in the formation of that which we know as our personal self. By now we have lived with that self for twenty or thirty years. We probably feel that we know it very well, inside and out.

Of course, by this time it will have been altered here and there, refined and deepened. There may have been important experiences—traumatic ones perhaps—which forced us to look again at who we were, or made us realize, looking back, that we had subtly changed. Bereavement, earthquake, war, sickness, travel, adventure, parenthood, promotion, there are many, many experiences which challenge us to change and grow, maybe a little, maybe a lot. Another one, and for many of us a big one, is menopause.

The type of challenge posed by menopause can often be a particularly comprehensive challenge. For many of us, it seems to be a challenge to review *everything*. At the very least, it creates a need for some reassessment. A reordering of priorities, maybe, or a reappraisal of our abilities and plans. Our children, if we have them, are probably gone or soon will be. Our work may be growing stale or changing. Younger people with ideas, ambitions, and endless energy may be crowding behind us on the career ladder. Do we keep going or retire? There are questions to answer, decisions to make. It is a time of stock-taking.

At the very most, menopause brings our entire world unglued. All the certainties of life are thrown into the melting pot at once. We can no longer feel sure of anything.

Your experience will be somewhere in between those two poles. Wherever it comes on that continuum, menopause is another vital one of those key life points in which we undertake, in some measure, a review of who we are.

I spoke in Chapter 3 about menopause as a challenge to our sense of who we are. At that point I was speaking primarily about who we *think* we are. As we have just discussed, there are both thinking and feeling components in the construction of our identities.

On the one hand you could say that our identities have been constructed as a result of millions upon millions of thoughts about the world and millions upon millions of decisions about how we want to play our part in that world, from moment to moment. As thinking creatures, we have to some extent consciously built an identity out of the feedback we have received from our environments and the decisions we have made with our minds.

On the other hand, since thinking and feeling are rarely found in isolation, our identities are in fact constructed from the interwoven fabric of both together. Our identity is built, not only from the conscious thoughts of our rational minds, but also from our historical collection of feelings—from the unconscious decisions, the ones which have taken place far below the level of our notice.

We are feeling creatures easily molded by emotional experience. There have been as many million experiences of feeling and emotion as there have of thought, and these have all gone into our shaping.

An image comes to mind of the techniques used to beat soft metal, such as copper or pewter, into pots and plates. Over and over, the tiny hammer beats on the surface of the metal, and gradually, the object changes shape. The repetitions of feelings and thoughts create their own patterns in the soft shape of our forming selves and gradually our identities evolve.

There is, however, another way which metal can be shaped, and that is by fire. Softened by the sudden intensity of heat, it will quickly bend. Then, when it cools, the shape is fixed. Thus can trauma heat us, and in the softness it creates, we are changed in shape. It has often been surmised that the earlier the trauma or the stronger the feelings, the greater is the intensity of the heat and the more drastic the result. A child who has been ill-treated or neglected in the early months of life may never learn to trust or love. A child who is raped may never be able to enjoy a normal sex life in adulthood.

These are extreme examples. However, for each of us there were fires in our childhood to a greater or lesser degree. For each of us there were strong feelings of some kind or another which left their mark on our psyches. The feelings of love and joy, comfort and pleasure created our likes and preferences; the feelings of fear and anger, repulsion and horror created our dislikes and phobias.

Many of these things we know and recognize, for we have discovered them at some time during our lives. But there may be many others which we do not know. There are experiences which we have forgotten and feelings which puzzle us, and sometimes these two sets of things connect. It is these forgotten feelings, awakened perhaps by a chance remark, which may pop up now in the increased sensitivity of menopause. It is these lost memories and repressed emotions which have created our cellar junk.

My daughter, in her late teens, came to me one day puzzled. She said, "I just turned the corner of the house and saw a magpie's feather in the rosemary bush. It gave me a strange, deep feeling of fear. Why on earth could that have been?"

I smiled and replied, "Don't you remember how frightened you were of feathers when you were little?"

"That's ridiculous!" she scoffed. "Why would anyone be afraid of feathers?"

I assured her it was true. As a toddler, she had gone through a phase of being scared to touch a feather. We never did discover why. In an attempt to desensitize her, I had stuck a magpie's feather in the wire mesh of the screen door so that she had to pass it many times a day, and over the months her fear decreased until at last she was able to touch the feather and finally to play with it.

The rosemary bush was right by that same door. Now, all those years later, a feather, blown by the wind, had lodged in the bush and she had rounded the corner and seen it there. Still engraved on her psyche was the faintest mark of the old fear. That was when I realized that nothing ever completely goes away. It merely fades to a faint trace.

This story illustrates another important discovery which most of us by now have made if we have been involved in any disciplines of self-awareness or personal growth. It is very simple. The first clue in solving any puzzle which remains within us is the awareness of an unexplained emotion or feeling. The tip-off may be—in fact it usually is—a reaction which does not quite make sense in the context in which it is felt. Why be scared of a feather? Likewise, why react with fury when our boss looks at us a certain way? When have we felt like that before? Was it at age five when we faced an angry parent or an unreasonable teacher? What are the feelings and beliefs within our five-year-old selves which remain buried within us to this very day? Old resentments, old fears, old formulations of the world—these are the building blocks of the reality we have created and in which, as adults, we live our lives, forever hiding, from others and ourselves, the truth of that little person within. Discovering the antecedents of our inappropriate behavior is a simple process. We have merely to notice the overreaction and then to ask ourselves, "What does this remind me of? When have I ever experienced this before?" If we relax and let our feelings lead us, they will unerringly lead us back to their own origins. This is how we set about cleaning the cellar.

I had been involved for many years in this kind of detection game of self-discovery. No doubt many of you will also be involved in it. Many forms of psychotherapy are based upon it; many self-help books are written about it. In those books and in the consulting rooms of all the therapists we can find 500 ways to trace the inner patterns and to change them.

There are books and therapies which encourage us to unearth the buried child and learn to love him or her. We are encouraged to discover our many selves, our top dogs and underdogs, our subpersonalities and our inner guides. We are urged to be O.K., heal our lives, love our disease, laugh, scream, love more, or not too much, relax, meditate, and affirm. There is a vast acreage of advice and expertise, all at our disposal. Theories and therapies of all kinds abound. Sometimes they conflict, and sometimes they say the same thing in different words and images. Sometimes it is bewildering.

What is your experience? I can only tell you mine. Maybe yours will be similar, maybe not. Maybe you can learn from mine, and maybe not. But at the very least, I believe that I can encourage you to keep exploring yours, whatever it is. I want to urge you to keep following your own unique path, reassured that it is, for you, the right one to be walking. Sometimes it may feel that it is not, but you must have faith that it is. If it were not, you would not be walking upon it.

But I do know bewilderment, and I do know doubt. I have often doubted. Doubt is natural. I am speaking of it here, for this is a book on menopause, and menopause, for me, brought some of the most severe doubts I had ever experienced. I began to doubt my confidence, my abilities, my sanity, my health, all the things I had taken for granted for so long.

I had read the books and done the courses, received the therapy, offered the therapy, taught the courses, made the changes, learned and grown and blossomed. I was getting

better and better, every day. Or so I believed. Then it started
to come undone. The undoing began when my menopause
began, and as menopause proceeded, so did the undoing. For
all my years of "growth" and all my successes at becoming
"better," there was nothing to show any more. I had begun
to spiral in toward the center, toward the vortex of despair
and emptiness.

* * *

It began with a dream. A dream that suddenly occurred
shortly after my fiftieth birthday.

The dream was of a woman, thin and still and ghostly pale.
In utter weariness and stillness, this woman in my dream was
lying, like a corpse, on a plain wooden gun carriage borne by
four spirited black horses.

The horses were snorting and their strong bodies were
glossy with sweat. The gun carriage moved across the night
sky, between the stars, and the woman lay still, unmoving,
being taken by the horses into some unguessed destiny.

As the entourage moved through the stars, there was thun-
der, lightning, and gunfire. The gun carriage was bombarded
with flying rocks and buffeted by cosmic winds of gale force.
The horses moved faster and faster. Eventually the woman,
together with the carriage and horses, was swept up into a
great whirlwind and broken into a million fragments.

As she began to disintegrate, the woman gave herself utterly
to the process and it became a dance. A dance of whirling
atoms. It became totally joyful and abandoned. All sense of
self was lost until there was just the dance and nothing else
existed in the universe.

Eventually, the great music faded and the dance slowed
down. Out of the shadows stepped the Goddess. She was tall,
much taller than a human woman, and indescribably beautiful. Her strength and energy were so vast that they filled up
the whole sky. She was dressed in robes so brilliant that one
could not look directly at them. She bent down. At her feet
was a tiny pile of multicolored fragments which had once
been the woman of the dream. The Goddess scooped up the
fragments and began to pour them into a brown paper su-

permarket sack. As the fragments ran through her fingers, it became apparent that each fragment was a jewel, a precious stone, which gleamed and twinkled in the reflected light from the eyes of the Goddess.

The dream ended when the sack was filled. There it sat, a neat little square parcel, all ready to be carried home.

* * *

This amazing and powerful dream was followed, a few days later, by the first hot flash, and then, over the ensuing months, by a whole series of dreams around the theme of dying mothers and a few more hot flashes.

Although my periods were still regular, I knew the dreams and the hot flashes were a signal that menopause was beginning. This was soon confirmed by my body when hot flashes began to happen regularly. Then the first missed period, and the physical process was underway.

The imagery of that wan, pale figure on the gun carriage stayed lodged inside me. It seemed to reflect what was happening to me. The robust figure I had made of myself was withering, somehow. My ego was eroding and the "topsoil" was washing away. I began to notice how my confidence was ebbing. It was as though all those affirmations had been for nothing, all that building of the new and "better" me had been merely an illusion. Fears I had overcome came back; doubts I had resolved returned. I felt as though I had triumphantly repelled some invading enemy horde only to find them still hiding in the garage! I began to fall into episodes of despair. That was when I discovered the cocoon.

At this time of our lives, many of us will need a cocoon. There is so much to deal with, and all the old ways of dealing with it seem to be failing us. We need a cocoon, in whatever form it may be available to us, in order to go inside in safety and in peace.

There are three stages to our task. First, we have to re-do all the work we have already done in understanding who we are. All those overreactions, all those neurotic fears, the traces of them are still there, no matter how well we have dealt with them in the past, and at this time of life they are likely to reemerge. Like the feather blown into the rosemary bush, seemingly trivial events may trigger old reactions we thought we had outgrown. It is as though all the important critical happenings in our lives have come up for review. Our childhood relationships with our parents, the identities we assumed for ourselves as teenagers and young adults, the sexual relationships with our partners, the plans and blueprints for our lives, all of it comes up for reconsideration. Like any other spring-cleaning, it takes some time to sort through it all. Time out—in the cocoon.

The second stage is when we realize that the particular set of reactions, neuroses, fears and phobias, personality characteristics, and so on which we have labeled "me," despite the few minor modifications and cosmetic improvements that we did manage to achieve, is basically as much an inevitable part of us as our unique personal package of now-aging skin and bones and internal organs. The little child that rides inside will be riding to the end of the line. She is not getting off after all. We are to be companions all the way. Just as no new sets of teeth will grow in our gums now, likewise no new psyche will replace the old one. The big change we have been waiting and striving for is never going to happen. This is it.

The third stage is the stage of accepting that this is O.K. and that it could not be any other way, and then learning to live out of that space of acceptance. That challenge may be the one that occupies us for the rest of our time on earth. May well be, in fact, for the further we progress into old age, the more we have to let go of the need to believe in the importance or centrality of those egoic "selves" which once were so important to us. The more we insist on keeping them central and seeing our lives through them, the harder it will be to relinquish them when the time comes, and the harder it will be to die in peaceful acceptance of our dying.

If we accept the challenge of reexamining the junk and cleaning the cellars of our unconscious minds, we may find a surprise hidden there. For in order to clean the cellar thoroughly, we have to go down into it. It is in that cellar that we have tossed the unwanted, repressed thoughts and feelings for all these years, and it is into that cellar that we must go

to find out what they all are. Not everyone finds the secret of
the cellar, but it is there, nonetheless.

When the cellar is swept clean—in other words, when we
have discovered as much as we can about the contents of our
own unconscious minds—its surprising secret is revealed. For
in the floor of that cellar is a trapdoor. And below the trapdoor
is a passage to another cellar. Only this other, deeper cellar,
rather than being below the foundations of our own house, is
as big and wide as the whole earth itself. It is the communal
cellar of all mankind. It is what Jung called the collective
unconscious.[1]

Our journeys, if we pursue them, will inevitably lead us
beyond the personal into the collective. In discovering our
hidden shadows, we discover the shadows of all mankind. By
personally accepting that unique human package that we are,
by ceasing to fight and strain against it and to attempt to
disown it and change it, we finally shoulder our full human
burden for the first time, consciously, knowingly, acceptingly,
lovingly. And in accepting the burden of our humanity in this
way, we symbolically shoulder the burden of all humanity,
as indeed Christ did. It is a profoundly redemptive act.

It is now that we realize that war does not start "out there,"
with the politicians; it starts in here, in our angry thoughts.
We realize that each one of us is capable of the sins of all. We
begin to realize that we are all one and that no one is going
anywhere without the rest. I shall speak further about this
communal aspect in Chapter 7.

Your experience will not necessarily be as I have outlined,
nor will it necessarily conform to the metaphors and images
generated by my mind in my attempts to describe what *I*
have felt.

Since we are, indeed, parts of the whole, there are often
fascinating similarities in our experiences. I have discovered
"dying mother" dreams in other menopausal women, for example, and also dreams and experiences of the Goddess.

The thoughts and feelings you encounter may be totally
different from any I have so far described. I do suspect,
though, that whatever process you find yourself in at this time
will be a potentially powerful one. I therefore offer you two

ideas which you may find useful. The first is the invitation to build a cocoon. The second is the idea of allowing yourself to spiral inward.

If possible, try to create some space in your life into which you can privately crawl to do your work. It may be that you need to maintain a busy life on the outside. If so, then reserve for yourself a separate time, however small, when there is absolutely nothing you need to do except go within and be with what is there. Even if it is only ten minutes a day, try to give it to yourself. You need, also, a quiet, undisturbed place if this is possible.

This is a time to examine your feeling-life, to see what is going on there, to hear and decipher the messages that are coming from inside.

If you are interested in exploring the opportunities of menopause, then now is the time. It is a perfect time to choose. You may care to start recording your dreams, if you are not already doing so, for they are rich sources of data about your unconscious processes. Rather than trying to analyze them, simply let them speak to you. Hold them lightly as you remember them, and let your mind play, rather than working with them. Free-associate to the images and symbols you find in your dreams rather than looking them up in books. In this way, you uncover your personal meanings rather than someone else's. If you need books to help you with your dreams, choose ones which amplify this way of working, such as Robert Johnson's *Inner Work*.[2]

Set aside some time for yourself, each day if possible. There are many creative ways you can use even small amounts of time. Any of them has the potential to take you further in your journey, to assist you in your inward spiral path toward the self. Here are some of them.

Dancing It Out

Moving the body—especially to music—can be for many people a powerful way of tuning in to the messages of the unconscious mind and liberating the feelings which have been locked inside the self, perhaps since babyhood. You may care to try this method of self-exploration.

Choose the time when you can be alone and have access to music and to a space large enough to dance in. The living room is usually fine.

You may find it advisable to start with some music which is fairly loud and has a heavy beat so that you stimulate and warm up your body with vigorous movement, getting your breathing going and your blood circulating freely. This also seems to liberate your inner energies. Dance as freely and as energetically as you can. Abandon yourself to the beat. Do this until you are warm and sweating and your body feels loose and full of energy.

Now choose some music which you would like to explore with movement. Preferably it should be instrumental rather than vocal and should be something which does not have fixed associations in your mind. It may be fast or slow, bright or subdued—whatever feels right in that moment of choosing. Let yourself be intuitively drawn toward a suitable piece of music and simply experiment with it. Put the music on and let yourself begin to move to it, without aim or purpose.

Simply express the sounds you hear through movement of your body. Since no one is watching, you are free to do whatever you like. Do not try to dance "properly" or to do any recognizable steps. Just move with the music, and without too much thought or plan. Let the music move *you* in whatever way it will. Drift with it. Dance your feelings. Dance your mood, your hopes, your fears. Dance your dread and your joy, your happiness, your worries. Dance your life, your experience, your pain, your journey. Dance your menopause. Dance it. Dance what menopause is, how it feels. Dance yourself. Eventually, the dance will reveal yourself to you and begin to release the bindings that have kept you prisoner. Dance yourself free. Dance it all.

Drawing It Out

This is a similar exercise to the "book cover" which we did in Chapter 1. However, this time, the object is to draw whatever you are feeling on this particular day, in this particular moment.

Once again, there is no need for artistic ability or for recognizable pictures. The aim of drawing our feelings is simply that. We put down, on the paper, whatever we are feeling at that moment.

Feelings may be expressed in stabs or smears of color, or they may be shapes and symbols, abstract patterns, or sketchy outlines. For myself, I find it helpful to have a large, spiral-bound sketchbook which I draw in from time to time with high-quality, colored, art pastels. I chose the pastels because they are a sensual delight to use. The pictures form a sort of diary of my feelings, from week to week. Often, I turn back to look at previous drawings, and new meanings appear; new insights arise as I see where I have been and what I was feeling in the light of what I am feeling now.

Singing It Out

For this, unless there is someone very close and trusted with whom you feel inclined to share the experience, it helps to be completely alone, preferably with the whole house to yourself. Even better, a deserted beach. Some people do this exercise in their cars, with the windows wound up, parked in a quiet spot somewhere. Walking alone in the country is also ideal. Anywhere you have the freedom to fill your lungs and sing, as loudly as you like.

It may help to begin with a recognizable song so that you can warm up your voice and get your breathing going. Then, without music and without thinking or planning, simply open your mouth and let your own sounds begin to emerge.

Sing your feelings. Sing your pain, your joy, your fear, your ideas. Sing how you are, who you are, right at this moment. Sing to your absent lover, to the children you bore or did not bear, to the dead and the living, to women and to men. Sing the naked truth of your heart, right now.

Tell the sky, the birds, the trees, the air around you. Let your song come out, without censoring or editing it. Simply sing. It does not have to have a rhythm or a melody. You may find your heart-song is a wail or a scream. Or it may be a soft hum. There may be words, in your own language or another. There may be only wordless sound.

Whatever it is, let it out. This is your song. Sing it to yourself so that you can hear it and know yourself. If you have emptiness, sing the emptiness. If there is confusion, sing the confusion. If you feel pain, sing out the pain. If there is joy, sing joy. If you find both, then sing both. Sing it all.

All of these exercises have the potential to arouse very deep emotions. It is therefore important to allow yourself time and space to express those emotions and, if necessary, to think about them and record them in your journal if you are keeping a journal. A journal at this time is also a useful tool. Writing down one's feelings helps to clarify and integrate them.

It is also important to create "buffer zones" around these times of exploration. You may need time to rest quietly for a while afterward, to take a shower, to read a few pages of a favorite book, or to do a meditation. You may need a cup of tea or a stroll in the garden, or even a nap. Whatever it is, allow time for it, so that you can then ease back into the business of your life.

These special times in the cocoon are your right. Grant them to yourself, fully; honor their importance, and never underestimate their potency.

5

TIME OF TRANSITION: THE COMMON THEMES OF MENOPAUSE

From time to time, in every person's life, there are major transitions to be made. These may result from crisis situations, such as bereavement, separation, illness, or injury, or from situational changes such as marriage, promotion, retirement, or travel.

Inevitably, there are also developmental transitions. Learning to walk is an important physical transition that almost everyone makes at an early age. Puberty can be a stormy transitional time. Menopause, too, is a transition, on many different levels.

West Coast psychologist William Bridges has been running courses and seminars since the early 1970s on the topic of life transitions. These courses are popular, since so many people find themselves struggling with the problems of transition phases in many different aspects of their lives. It is useful to know something of the theory of life transitions. I have found Bridges' work invaluable in helping me to make sense of menopause.[1]

Bridges has pointed out that there appears to be a common structure underlying all transitions, regardless of the category into which they fall, situational or developmental. This structure is a three-part one.

Every transition, says Bridges, begins with an ending. For any change to happen, there is first something which has to end. For a child to walk, there has to be an end to the satisfaction with crawling as a routine method of locomotion. For a human being to become adult, there has to be an end to childhood. Even though the new may be glimpsed, the old has to be put away before the new can become the norm. In many transitions, particularly the crisis ones, it is the sudden end of something—a death, an accident, a retrenchment at work, a partner leaving—which heralds the transition, and the new beginning is not even glimpsed until the ending has happened.

Between the ending and the new beginning, there is a third place. That is the place which Bridges calls "the neutral zone." It is the place in which our hearts and minds dwell as we do all the necessary work involved with endings and beginnings. It is a vital stage in most processes of transition. It may be long or short. It may take years or minutes.

Sometimes we are fully aware of what is ending and what is beginning and what needs to be done. At other times, we seem to be stuck, lost in a fog, uncertain of our direction. We may not even know what the new will be, nor even clearly understand what has ended, what has to be let go or completed. The neutral zone may feel like depression. We may feel alienated from the past and not yet connected to the future. It may seem like limbo.

I have found this three-stage way of viewing transitions a very useful one in the study of menopause. As menopausal women, we are all working through a transition process.

This is taking place on the physical plane, as our bodies reach the end of their reproductive phase and prepare for a new existence with drastically reduced levels of hormones.

On a mental and emotional level, we are adjusting to a new way of thinking and feeling, a new definition of ourselves as nonfertile women whose ways of being in the world and contributing to it are no longer tied to the possibility of creating children. We may also be concurrently involved in other transition processes which have a bearing on these definitions. Our children may be leaving home or our parents may have become infirm or be dying. Our careers may have peaked and be starting the gentle wind-down toward retirement or we may in fact have chosen early retirement and be facing the massive lifestyle transition which can come with that.

Spiritually, we are likely to be in the transitional phase of which Jung spoke, a turning away from our preoccupation with the outer world of the ego and a beginning of the inner journey of exploration, the journey toward the true self and what lies beyond it.

So menopause itself may be seen as one big transition phase. It may feel like many years spent in the neutral zone dealing with endings and wondering if there are any new beginnings beyond it. Or it may be a period of time during which the changes happen but we do not really notice them until long after they have happened. For some women preoccupied with the outer details of their lives, these processes take place below the threshold of awareness. For them it is a source of puzzlement to find that other women have been bogged down in any way by menopause. They are the ones whose major challenges lie elsewhere, and for them this book may not seem relevant at all. That is all as it should be. We do not all choose the same path, and there is richness in our vast variety.

At first, in my studies of menopause, I was puzzled to find what appeared to be such contradictory evidence. There did appear to be certain recurring themes and issues which many women spoke about, and yet they spoke about them in such different, and sometimes diametrically opposite, ways that it seemed extremely confusing. Furthermore, when I first applied the theory of transitions to the stories and experiences which these women recounted, it was hard to determine, in many cases, whether an individual woman was experiencing an ending, a beginning, or a neutral zone.

Then I realized that menopause is not simply one big transition. It is also a set of smaller transitions within the big one. Once I realized that, everything fell into place. I could see that each woman was dealing with a set of issues and was dealing with them in a certain order. One issue may have been resolved and another is only just being discovered. So, questioned about one aspect of menopause, such as the end of fertility, she may be deep in grief, whereas on another issue, such as the question of physical appearance, she may feel completely at ease with the aging process. Another woman may be wrestling with the agony of her wrinkles and yet delighted to be through with childbearing. A third may have resolved all these emotional issues and yet be plagued by physical symptoms which cause her so much discomfort that she turns to medicine for relief, such as the woman who told me she had to change her entire bed linen every night, so badly did she sweat.

Let me share with you now the six main themes which seem to be the most common ones for the menopausal women I know and have known. These may or may not be personal issues for you or for other women with whom you are connected, but I suspect that they are issues to which you have given at least a little thought if you are in the menopause stage of your life.

The first of these themes is the one I have named "Biology as Destiny." The issues here are the issues of femininity. This is where we examine our attitudes to being female and living in a female body, with its female rhythms and its potential for the creation and birthing of new life.

BIOLOGY AS DESTINY

As we saw in Chapter 2, there are some women who abhor the menstrual cycle and some who revel in it. There are others who are neutral or ambivalent about it. Likewise, some women dislike childbearing, others delight in it, and some are neutral or ambivalent.

Not surprisingly, therefore, these same differences appear in women's attitudes regarding the end of their reproductive cycles. When I asked questions about these issues I found that women who had disliked having periods were delighted that menstruation was ceasing. Nevertheless, for some of them, this definitive sign of the ending of their fertility created ambivalence and the need to work through issues of relinquishing the motherhood role or its potential.

This was an issue whether they had had children or not. For those who had not, it meant relinquishing an option or a dream, even if it were an option they had chosen not to exercise, or, for infertile women, a dream which had always been hopeless. Pauline, a successful career woman who had long since decided to remain childless, began softly crying in our women's group one day. "I thought that was all over and done with," she said, through her tears, "but now I realize it is all still there." On a rational level, her decision was history. But the emotions of menopause had revealed to her that on another level, the issue was still very much alive, and would have to be thought about, felt about, cried about some more maybe, before it could be laid to rest with finality.

I remember, too, the anguished sobs of Julia, whose approaching menopause heralded the end of a long-held fantasy. From years of endometriosis, her Fallopian tubes were totally blocked and natural conception was, for her, out of the question. Furthermore, because her partner suffered from a chronic psychiatric condition and could not cope with pressure, she had passed up the option of taking part in an in vitro fertilization (IVF) program that the doctor warned would be stressful for both partners. The couple was interviewed by an adoption agency but not considered suitable as adopting parents. Julia made her career in child care and resigned herself to the fact that she could never be a biological mother. Yet deep inside her, the fantasy lived on. The hoped-for miracle never came, but each month, when her period started, she would think to herself, "Maybe next month it will happen." The hormonal swings of beginning menopause brought more gynecological problems and Julia's specialist recommended a hysterectomy.

"It was like I shut all the grief away in a cupboard," she said. "Now the door of the cupboard is open and I can't get it shut again. The tears just won't stop."

They did stop, eventually, but only because she let them flow until the cupboard was emptied. Then there was peace. Julia was able to move on.

For those whose families were long since complete, there was still the need to redefine themselves as women who could bear no more children, even if they had wanted to do so. This is different from simply not having any more babies. It has finality. An open invitation is no longer. A door is locked and bolted. Even if it were a door through which you had never again intended to walk, there is still a certain shock in finding it firmly bolted against you, permanently. Anne has several grown-up children, and no intention of starting again. And yet, when asked to write her thoughts about menopause, she wrote, "I have struggled with the meaning of my life if I can no longer bear children...it is final, like death. On the one hand I don't want to raise a child and on the other I still have some yearnings."

Bernice, who has never had children and has never wanted any, is a lesbian. For her, menopause has meant that with her ability to produce children has gone her last chance of earning her stripes in that world of "respectability" which has never understood nor honored her sexuality. For her, there is a bitterness in it, as well as a sadness.

Jungian analyst Ann Mankowitz made and published a study of menopause as experienced by one of her analysands, a woman named Rachel who revealed her process in a series of dreams. The dreams were filled with vivid imagery, which yielded up its meanings in therapy, enabling Rachel to work through the key issues of her life change. "There is an enigmatic significance about the loss of reproductivity," remarks Mankowitz, "that cannot be denied or explained away." Rachel, she tells us, "had all the children she wanted and for years she had been actively preventing more births, yet she felt grief at her involuntary and perpetual barrenness, as if at a personal bereavement." By taking the time to listen to her dreams and to work through them with her therapist, Rachel was able to complete her mourning process and begin to embrace her new freedom. "What she had mourned was her own *fruitfulness*: the very word seems to make the grieving understandable, in spite of all the rational denial."[2]

Women who have taken delight in their menstrual rhythms, even though they may have found the practicalities of menstruation burdensome, often mourn the cessation of that known, expected rhythm. And again we find ambivalence. As one woman explained it,

> I have mixed feelings. I am in the midst of changes. Instead of regularity I have no schedule and never know from month to

month what will happen. At times I find this a bit unsettling, at others I am pleased to find that changes are taking place. I don't mind not having the fuss of tampons, napkins, and so on. So there is both a sense of freedom and a sense of something familiar lost.

Something familiar is indeed lost, irrevocably. The rhythm we have lived with for so long is gone forever. Whether we have admitted it into consciousness or not, one of the transition tasks of menopause is to mourn this loss on a symbolic level. As Mankowitz explains it,

> That phrase, "gone forever," brought home to me again the symbolic significance of the end of fertility. As well as the actual conceptions, pregnancies and births that may have shaped the realities of her life, the woman of fifty has lived for thirty-five years or more with the monthly repetition of the potential to create new life. Whatever her conscious attitude or her unconscious reactions toward this cycle, it inevitably represents the constant power of renewal. At menopause that power ceases, and to the menopausal woman it seems at first that hope has gone forever, it is too late, the future is empty.
>
> As the end of a lifelong rhythm, then, the change of life requires of her that she learn to live from day to day and rediscover her creativeness in a new direction. That is the task and that is the future.[3]

We must remember, of course, that menopause itself is not the only trigger that sets off the fertility issue. One woman explained to me that she had had to resolve this many years previously, when deciding on a tubal ligation. For her, therefore, it was a task long since completed. She entered her major transition of menopause with one minor transition already made.

Sometimes, the recognition of these emotional issues occurs before any physical signs have manifested and is actually the first signal that menopause is happening. A woman who thought that she had dealt with many of the issues before menopause described to me the big "crunch" that she had experienced on her fiftieth birthday. That day was a crisis point for her and she began to face and to work through all the issues we are now discussing. Menopause itself, at that time, had not come to her notice physically, nor had it come into her consciousness that she was indeed entering the menopause process, as we have defined it here. Her fiftieth birthday can be seen, in fact, as her entry point into menopause, albeit unrecognized as such. For many of us, I believe, the beginning is a subtle psychic event which we do not necessarily see for what it is. My own menopause began with my dream of the pale woman on her journey through the night sky. That point might have gone unnoticed had I not been so keen to explore the deeper meanings of the dream and had it not been followed by a noticeable, physical sign of change.

The second recurrent theme, and one to which almost every menopausal woman I have met has alluded, is the one I think of as "Fading Roses." Here we find the twin issues of physical appearance and sexuality.

FADING ROSES

Why is there such a strange pain that comes to some of us as we contemplate that changing face in the glass?

Elissa Melamed in her book *Mirror, Mirror: The Terror of Not Being Young* speaks poignantly of the psychic battle that for many women seems to underlie the apparently simple facts of physical aging.

> I realize that I was obviously dealing with something deeper than some wrinkles and grey hairs. I was feeling divided, divided against myself: a changeless person trapped inside a changing body; a centered person at odds with a needy person; an honest person ashamed of the "me" who wanted to play the youth game.[4]

In our youth-oriented society, "good looks" and juicy sexuality are currency. It is not surprising, therefore, that many women dread the day when they will have nothing to sell in the market but a set of wrinkles and a dry vagina.

Many of the women whom I have questioned have seemed, like Elissa Melamed, transfixed and perplexed by their changing reflection in the mirror and in men's eyes. One said that she wished she could retain the feelings of freedom she has now, but also be twenty-five years old again. So here we begin to see another ambivalence. There is often a conscious pleasure in one's feelings of maturity, which lies side by side with a conscious anxiety about one's changing image from youthfulness to middle age, and the resultant effect on one's sexual self and relationships.

As with all ambivalence, there is a time when we are balanced midway between the two poles and can feel no movement. This is in the nature of many transitions. The neutral zone frequently feels like a stuck place. But imperceptibly, as time passes, there is the awareness of a subtle shift. If we are prepared to stay with ambivalence, rather than trying to force ourselves into feeling either one way or the other, then gradually we move, until one day we find that the scales have settled down on one side or the other and we are at peace.

Joan, a nurse in her late forties, spoke to me of that shift as she experienced it in her life. "There has been a lot of emotional grieving for the loss of my younger, sexier-looking self," she explained, "but also a feeling of liberation from having to maintain that image." Once we have been able to relinquish our own inner concept of our bodies as perpetually young and nubile, there is suddenly the freedom simply to live in them, to dress for comfort, to relax.

In speaking with Joan, one can feel that she is coming toward a resolution of that issue now. It comes through in her very words. However, Joan does have a permanent partner, a man she has lived with for many years and with whom she has a particularly good sexual relationship. How much harder is it for women to negotiate this particular hurdle when they are sexually alone and wish they had partners?

For heterosexual women, who are the majority, I believe it can be particularly difficult. Since we are all conditioned into a game of sexual competition where youth holds all the best cards, it takes a strong woman to maintain her feeling of inner

beauty when the mirror and men's eyes are beginning to dis-
count her. Listen to the words of a woman for whom this is
the central issue of menopause right now:

> I do feel the stigma of being an aging female. I feel so much
> stronger and wiser and yet I can't help but be affected by the
> cult of youth. Since I'm single and would like to find a mate
> I'm aware of my low marketability because of my age. I think
> if I were in a stable marriage this aspect of aging would not
> be so hard. For me menopause is just a symbol of aging.

Had she compared her feelings with the next speaker, however, she might have discovered that even within a relationship the issues of looks and sexuality may still be
problematical.

Melanie describes herself as happily married. There was a
rocky time in her marriage some ten years ago, but the issues
were resolved. In the resolving, Melanie and her husband,
Rob, discovered a deeper intimacy than they had ever experienced before, and these days they seem to be even more
deeply in love then ever they were. Melanie has made a particular study of color and fashion, and in the years since the
children left and money became more available, she has paid
particular attention to her wardrobe, her figure, and her
health. Rob has responded with delight and pride in her appearance, which is both youthful and elegant.

Yet when we spoke of menopause, Melanie revealed some
doubts and fears. She said that she was finding herself making
comparisons, these days, between herself and her younger
colleagues at work and beginning to feel left out. It was as
though they all belonged to some invisible club from which
she, by virtue of her age, was now excluded.

Not only that, but her libido was changing, and this worried
her. She mused: "periods of a lack of sexual urge make me
wonder whether that rich part of my life will ever be the same.
So there is some anxiety attached to how I will feel about
myself as a woman afterwards."

For so many of us, then, the physical appearance of our
bodies and the way we express our sexuality are crucial issues

which must be considered during the menopausal transition time.

We must make decisions. Do we wish to maintain an active sex life well into old age? If so, how do we feel about displaying our aging body to another? If the other is one who has long known and loved us and our body, there is probably no problem, but what if we seek a new partner, like the single woman quoted above?

Our logical minds may tell us that love is a holistic thing and that we care only to be loved for who we are and not for how young we are or look. Yet the popular culture dances to a different song, whose lyrics may sound cruel to our ears. Not because our culture is in any sense "wrong" but because our culture is only the human version of any other culture in any other species. The young, nubile females are sexually attractive to the males; the old, infertile ones less so. It is a biological imperative with obvious benefits to the healthy continuation of any species. It is Nature, as she is, honest and ruthless. When we see it, really see it, we can laugh. When we can laugh at the honesty and the reality of it, and at ourselves, we have completed that transition. Then we can love our own aging bodies and smile at the fading rose petals in the mirror. We can even start to glimpse another, different kind of beauty in ourselves. But until then, it can hurt a lot.

Some of the decisions may be practical. To make love, it helps to have a vagina which is fleshy and wet, yet as our estrogen production wanes, the lack of this hormone causes the tissue within the walls of our vaginas to become thinner and dryer. In coitus, this can lead to considerable discomfort. Can we make do with lubricating gel or do we need to use an estrogen-based cream or even to decide that this is an indication for hormone replacement therapy?

If the emotional issues of menopause do not surface of their own accord, sometimes the practical decisions such as these will force their emergence for us.

At fifty-one I stopped wearing makeup. That, for me, was the turning point. It was the point at which I let myself really look into the mirror and feel the pain. It had been thirty years since I had gone out into the street without at least some makeup on, and I had always felt that I looked insignificant and plain without it. Now I forced myself to reexamine those old feelings.

Instead of continuing the denial that went with lipstick and eye shadow, I faced the full reality of my face and began to deal with the issues on a deeper level. My decision to stop wearing makeup was a symbol that I had accepted the challenge and was working through it. For some people, such an action might have been unnecessary, but for me it was the only way to break through my own resistance. It was as though I grabbed myself by the arm and threw myself against the mirror, saying, "Look, there it is, your face. It is getting old. *You* are getting old. Face it!"

This theme of "Fading Roses" is almost certainly a key one for many women, as it has been for me. And because of the inventions of modern science, it is tied up with the next theme, which is the theme of "Medicalization."

THE MEDICALIZATION OF MENOPAUSE

There is no doubt that hormone replacement therapy does delay the physical effects of aging inasmuch as it replaces the lost estrogen, and estrogen is an important preserver of skin tone, hair luster, vaginal elasticity, and so on.

It is also an undeniable fact that hormone therapy reduces a woman's risk of osteoporosis, heart disease, and various other illnesses. It has brought other problems in its wake, as we know, and this has made many women wary of embarking on it.

However, because of the huge potential market for a perfected version, medicine is working hard and fast toward perfecting the still-controversial therapy. It is likely that at some time in the near future we shall have the option of a "treatment" that safeguards us against the postmenopausal health risks while being guaranteed free of unwanted side effects. The question is, should we take it?

Each woman will have to decide this for herself. I have been struggling with *my* answer.

My fear is that by turning menopause from a stage of life into a medical condition we shall lose more than we shall gain.

If menopause becomes a medical condition from which we all seek a "cure," then yes, it can give us more years of the same quality of life that we enjoyed in our thirties, maybe. But is that what we deeply want?

Is there not some part of us, some biological clock inside us, that triggers the right challenges at the right times? Is there not a part of our psyche that intuitively knows when it is time to be considering the important questions and themes of change? In "curing" or at least "alleviating" our "condition," do we run the risk of losing something very important about our experience of being female? Is it not the deep female within us that understands and accepts the cyclic nature of all existence just as she experiences the cyclic nature of herself?

Symbolized in Hindu culture by the Goddess Kali, with her neck adorned with skulls and her fangs dripping blood, the female is not only the carrier of cyclicity in life but also the one who reminds us of the cyclicity of all things, and that means the inevitability of death. The deep female in us does not shrink from the knowledge of death. She is there to remind others of it. She does not go out to fight it like the heroic male. She celebrates it as a part of life, for life includes death. Old age and death. Winter, spring, summer, and fall. The female is whole and knows all the parts. She is the carrier of cyclicity, the one who does not let us forget.

Menopause is the fall, and precedes the winter of old age and death. Fall prepares us for winter. The leaves fall and the trees stand bare. The cold days come gradually. There is a need for fall. So, too, there may be a need for menopause.

Am I being reactionary and conservative or am I tapping into a deep truth?

So many questions, and each of us must consider them for herself and be true to herself in the answering.

This brings us to the fourth theme. I have called it "Rehearsal for Death."

REHEARSAL FOR DEATH

The woman on the gun carriage was going to her death in a way. Yet she was not killed but rearranged. You could say that none of us is ever more than rearranged. It is certainly true in a basic, physical sense. Our parts are endlessly recycled, for that is the nature of life on earth. Our bodies die and rot, breaking down into raw material from which new life-forms are eventually constructed. The carbon atoms that form the raw material of these hands I see before me will one day be part of a frog or a crocus, a ladybug maybe, or a patch of lichen on a rock.

Most species seem to accept these facts quite comfortably. Humanity is less comfortable about them. Each human being has a consciousness that appears to bring, almost inevitably, a troubled awareness of his or her mortality. So for most of us, there seems to be a need to come to terms with dying; the need to resolve what the fact of death means to us, personally and collectively.

It helps to rehearse, and menopause is a way of rehearsing. There are so many little deaths. Each of the separate transitions is a little death in itself. The acceptance of one's fading "looks," the end of fertility, the loss of one's natural hormones, and the consequent decision about whether to accept that or to start the replacement therapy, all these are transitional issues. Each is a little death, in its own way, of some aspect of the known, familiar self we have lived with so long. It is a precious opportunity, peculiar to women, this opportunity to rehearse for the final performance of our lives, for the death which will inevitably come.

My dreams, at the start of menopause, were all about the death of the mother. Since my particular identity in the preceding years had been crystallized around motherhood, the end of my active mothering phase was indeed a little death for me. The end of wearing makeup and seeing myself in terms of the currency of the youth culture, that was another little death. It was the death of my self-image as a sex object even though in my own eyes I had always been a flawed one.

For the women who shared their experiences with me, death

was a theme which ran deeply through their words and the pictures they drew for me. If often manifested itself in the commentaries which they added to their drawings.

Women spoke to me of the inner urge to complete things left unfinished, the need to put one's house in order, both physically and metaphorically. Some said that now, at menopause, they were consciously thinking more about death and how they would deal with it when it came to them.

The loss of parents was also involved here, for some women, as a stimulus which brought these issues up for consideration. One woman reflected that, with the aging of her parents, she was now aware of becoming part of the generation that is "next in line."

As she said that, I had a vivid image of a game we used to play at school when I was very small. It was a variety of tag which we called "Twos and Threes." We stood in pairs, one behind the other, forming an inward-facing circle. Around and between the circle and the pairs, two children chased each other. To escape, the one being pursued could join on the back of any pair, at which point the one in front had immediately to leave and become the target. It felt so much safer to be the one at the back. I remember so vividly the feeling which came to me—the panic of imminence—as the person in front of me suddenly ran away and I became the next in line with nothing but open space in front of me, waiting.

For many women, a diffuse awareness of the cyclicity of life—the eternal succession of generations, whether of leaves on the trees or of humans in families—seems to be a backdrop to their menopausal experience and a way of giving it meaning and relaxing into it. One woman quoted the 119th Psalm— "a time to love and a time to die"—and another looked down the hollow tube of the future and saw "my children, their children, their children's children." Others quoted the seasons. One person said, "Women are like relay races. You come to the end of your stretch and you pass the baton on to one of your daughters (if you have one) to continue with her daughter until it is her turn to pass it on." Another quoted Homer: "As is the generation of leaves, so is that of humanity."

It is woman who tends the entrances and exits of life. She

gives birth and assists at birthing and often ministers to the sick and dying. A woman knows the seasons of life deep inside her cyclic nature. Menopause, it seems to me, is her time to reflect upon these truths and to rediscover the death which is inherent in all life. When she has come to terms with the autumn colors of her own life, she is more fully woman.

These discoveries, these themes, these workings-through, all of them are part of the whole process which Jung called individuation. It is the process of discovering and building the someone that we are and then learning to let go of the need to be someone. It is a spiraling inward to the core of our being, wherein resides the self. From there, the spiraling inward can change to a magnificent and radiant spiraling outward. This inward journey is the fifth of my key themes. I shall speak of it in the next chapter.

Meanwhile, I should like you to consider the transition process in relation to your own life.

* * *

Take a look at what is ending or has ended. Have you completed your endings? Have you done your grieving for that which can never return? Until we deal with our endings we cannot proceed to our new beginnings.

Take stock of where you are as regards each of the issues we have discussed in this chapter. Think about the end of your lifetime of menstruation, the end of your fertility. How do you feel about your physical appearance? Have you considered all the pros and cons of hormone replacement therapy and come to a decision on that issue? What is your attitude to death?

A note of warning. If you find yourself scoffing about any of these issues, this may be a sign that you have not in fact resolved it but have repressed it. If it is truly resolved inside you, the feeling will be one of recognition and of quiet compassion for those who have not yet resolved it.

Maybe you have that foggy feeling of being in the neutral zone. There may be no clear idea of what is approaching, no sense of purpose or direction. You may feel a sense of ambivalence about some of the issues. That is perfectly natural and normal. Have the patience to stay with your ambivalence for as long as it takes. Rather than worrying at the issues like a tongue returning to a sore tooth, simply let them rest for a while. This is the time to snuggle down inside the cocoon, feel your hot flashes, and let the process simply happen. It is like gestation or pupation, a natural process of creation, and it cannot be hurried.

Our only obligation is to deal with our endings and await our new beginnings with patience and expectancy. Not by having rigid expectations as to how they should be, but awaiting them patiently, openly, ready to greet them whatever they are, as we greet a newborn child, with a welcome.

6

WHO AM I REALLY?

One of the major themes of menopause is the theme of individuation. Individuation, you will remember, is a Jungian term describing the process by which each individual human being unfolds and develops, becoming steadily more and more who he or she is.

When I think of the word "individuation," particularly as it is applied to this stage of life, there is a sense of deepening, a sense of ever-increasing richness, like the maturing of fine wine. The potential in the bud spreads out under the sun to become a flower, and beyond the flower there is the fruit. Menopause may be the beginning of the harvest, the first taste of the ripening fruit.

Unlike the other transition processes of which we have spoken, the process of individuation can come to no completion before death, since it is by definition a journey which lasts a lifetime. The transition task of menopause, therefore, is not the individuation process itself, since that is a process which begins at conception and continues to death. Rather, I see our task as bringing the process, perhaps for the first time, into full, conscious awareness.

Once we are aware, we are on our way. This is the completion we are seeking. The ending is the ending of unconsciousness, of blindly following a scripted role—albeit one we may ourselves have scripted—and beginning the search for who we are inside. It is the ending of that automatic way of living where we left no room for reflection, no room for contemplation of the deeper self. It is the ending of that busyness which kept our focus on outer tasks, with doing things in the world, in whatever form that took for us. For many of us, those were tasks which kept us preoccupied with the needs of others, whether at home or at work. For many, it involved a priority system that invariably put us last on the list. Our self-nurturing and self-exploration, if they existed at all, were marginal to the main business of life, which was outer-focused, task-centered, and frequently involved overriding our deeper needs and patterns, our inner rhythms and cycles.

For some women, at this time of life the outer tasks themselves may begin to change, forcing awareness. Outer changes may be forced upon us by circumstance. Like the first cold winds of October, they may herald the approach of a time that is different, a time of less frantic outer activity, a time of in-turning.

When the nest empties, and child voices around the house are but remembered echoes, there is a quietness which descends. At first, in that quietness there may be depression, a cold grayness that blocks out the grief, the fear, and the sense of change and challenge, in the same way that a cloud blocks the energy of the sun. But it is into those blocked feelings that we must go. Into the grief, into the challenge, into the fear that change so often brings.

In the new quietness, there is a chance to be, at last, face to face with the self.

So often women react to the imposed changes, such as the empty nest, with unthinking panic and rush to find replacements for their lost tasks. They search frantically for substitute ways to use up their time and energy on outer-focused activity, seeking to replicate the patterns and routines of the era that is ending. Many books on menopause encourage this. One male doctor, an acknowledged "expert" on menopause, exhorts his readers, "You must do something. You must enjoy it. Above everything else, GET INVOLVED."[1] Not for his patients the cocoon.

Women are told they must do something, anything, as long

as it keeps them busy and occupied and feeling useful. Rarely are we encouraged simply to sit and be. To sit and be with what is happening within. To go inside and encounter all that which has been waiting for such an opportunity as this.

This is the "neutral zone" in the menopausal stage of individuation. It is where we sit, quietly, until we can feel what has ended, what is ending, and, finally, what is beginning.

What is beginning is a new era. It is an era in which we shall use our time and energy differently. We shall begin to nurture and explore the self as a mainstream activity rather than as a hobby that fits around the edges of an other-centered lifestyle. The activities we undertake in the world, whatever they are, will be ones which grow naturally out of our appraisal of ourselves and our growth patterns. They will be activities we choose, projects which grow out of the humus of our creative minds as we allow ourselves time to germinate the seeds of them. They will be projects and activities important to our hearts, not time-fillers randomly grabbed to fill a space, like magazines in a dentist's waiting room or a novel hastily purchased from the airport newsstand. They will be activities and projects which grow from us, from who we deeply are. We shall not need to run in desperate search of them.

The ending is the gradual cessation of much that has defined our lives in the so-called "productive" years. The neutral zone is where we are lost. There may be a feeling of coming undone, of wondering what is happening to us. Our ship of security is sinking and we are trying to stay afloat in a sea of inner change. The beginning is our conscious embrace of the individuation process.

Some women reject the call to enter the cocoon of self-exploration on the basis that it is simply an exercise in self-centered navel-gazing. Trained to believe that their focus should be on helping others, they cannot bear to take time for self-discovery. It is my strong belief—and my personal experience bears testimony to this—that the opposite is true. The true goal of self-discovery, if that process is pursued to its limits, is the transcendence of the personal, egoic self altogether. A woman who has made this journey through the cocoon and come out at the other end will no longer be focused on her personal, individual concerns but will be a child of the collective. She will have cleaned her own cellar and discovered the trapdoor that connects her to the whole. The goal of the individuation process is not selfishness but an eventual moving beyond the individual self altogether and a coming to know the true self, the deepest layer of being which, in a simplified way, one could describe as the soul of us all.

The way to it, however, is down and in and through. We must discover who we are before we can release it—or if you like, before it releases us.

The women whose menopausal experience I have studied are all clearly manifesting this dawning of awareness of their own processes of individuation. Many are still in the throes of discovering their true identities beneath the roles they have dutifully performed and within which they may have become lost as unique individuals. Over and over again, the message seems to be, "Now is the time for *me*."

There can be few among us today who are altogether unfamiliar with this theme, for the whole matter of woman's loss of personal identity has been a central issue in feminist thinking and writing for several decades now. Many researchers have asked women about the midlife era of change and self-discovery. Lillian Rubin, for example, is a researcher who interviewed many women in the menopausal age group. Numbers of them were making the step to self-discovery after half a lifetime of performing prescribed roles and they spoke about it with deep feeling.[2] In many such studies, the focus has been on the practicalities, the reactions of others, the rearrangement of time and energy. I have tried to go even deeper, searching for the growth in inner awareness and the consciousness of the individuation journey.

As Jung said, the afternoon of life has a significance of its own and the proper focus of this period is that journey inward, towards the self. For women who have spent many years locked into motherhood or career roles which defined the parameters of their identities and absorbed each daily ration of energy, now it is time to begin the inner search. I have tried to see how deep that search was going. For me, it has gone very deep, deeper than I had ever been before. I wanted to know how deeply it was going for others. That was when I began to research the experience of other menopausal women and to find that many of their experiences paralleled my own.

Women spoke of their increased assertiveness, their heightened sense of purpose, their determination to carve out time for their own pursuits, their quest to find out who they were as individuals. They also spoke of their pain and lostness, their sense of endings and beginnings, and the confusion that is the neutral zone.

For some this may be the first time—at least since adolescence—that they have pondered so introspectively and searched for answers to life's deeper questions. It may feel like a change of personality. Take, for example, Marie, who is now fifty-four. She wrote for me this summary of her menopause process:

> I felt I changed from a person who just worked from 6 A.M. to 10 P.M. to someone who was able to sit and question why. Gradually I felt more confident in demanding time for my own interests and work instead of being a wife and mother first and leaving little or no time for self. For a while I was pretty depressed whilst I went through that sorting and reassessing process. It sure rocked the boat at home!

Marie had brought up a large family. Her husband had become an invalid, retiring from work at the same time that her teenage children, needing guidance in their various encounters with the world beyond home, turned to their mother with their personal crises. She was the anchor for them all. Meanwhile, her career as a health educator was blossoming and creating more demands on her time and energy. For a while she tried to do it all. As menopause kicked in, with its days of lethargy, cotton-head, and chaotic feelings, Marie entered a time of crisis. The change of which she speaks, the change which made of her "someone who was able to sit and question why," took several years. Now, she looks back and can see the process in retrospect. Out now from the other end of her fog, Marie feels good about herself. She has passed through the neutral zone. She is exploring new beginnings, and with a new zest.

Soula's experience has been somewhat different. The same age as Marie, Soula was brought up in another culture, where female individuation has traditionally been more difficult than in my own. She, too, married a man whose health was poor and whose demands on her increased at the same time that the children were becoming adult and the physical facts of menopause were manifesting. She, too, felt the same urges to individuation, the inner promptings to find out who she was, beyond the wife and mother and career roles. However, in speaking of these urges to me, Soula referred to them as "selfish thoughts." Her longing for the freedom to explore was condemned by her culture, speaking as an inner voice, calling her "selfish" for wanting to find herself as an individual. She was hesitant, fearful, and slightly bitter, too. For her an inner war was raging. To follow the call to individuation meant defying an internalized cultural taboo.

There are many women who display a slight air of bravado or defensiveness when speaking of their individuation process; for example, "I have looked after others for years. Now it is *my* turn." As though this were something to be earned rather than a general human birthright.

I have discovered, however, that there are many for whom it has been a journey embarked upon with gusto and a sense of adventure. In their speaking, writing, and drawing, the word "freedom" has come up over and over again. Like Catherine, who said, "Most of the time there is a feeling of freedom and of space and time into which I can move. I know I am me. A year ago I would have said, 'I am the mother of three children and....' " For most of us, the turbulence of menopause throws up old issues for reexamination. If we allow it to, that is. "Who am I?" is not a question that is easily tackled, let alone easily resolved. As in adolescence, the struggle of identity can be a painful one. For a woman who has lived many years dressed in the costume of mother, wife, homemaker, or various career identities, to stand naked again and ask "Who am I really?" is to invite an unaccustomed degree of vulnerability, perhaps even terror. Several women spoke of "breakdowns." Another drew a poignant picture, in pen and ink, of a woman standing naked in a busy city street. "That", she said, "is how I feel."

It is the artwork which has shown me, where often words could not, the depth of exploration which is happening within the women who have shared with me, and the intensity of feelings, both negative and positive. Black clouds, tornadoes, tunnels, rainbows, blood-red flowers. So many wonderful images. Pain and joy, conflict and clarity, struggle, breakdown, and breakthrough. So much rich experience.

Claire drew the outline of an egg, its shell breaking, the woman bursting out. Menopause, she said, is the process of breaking out. "During a woman's productive years, it is as though she is inside a cage with definite limitations. Menopause is like the birthing of a new woman—one who can be or do anything she wants to. No society expectations." That is Claire's menopause, a celebration of freedom. In her drawing, the woman who emerges from the egg is wearing a huge smile, and next to her the words, "Free at last!"

The vast and rich variety of experience that reveals itself as I ask and probe into the lives of my contemporaries is a constant source of delight to me. Likewise, the twin sister of that delight is the comfortable knowledge that we have a commonality of experience, as women, that forever unites us, not only with each other but with all women living, dead, and unborn.

It is tempting, out of this delight in our similarities, to search for generalizations. There is a certain comfort in knowing that we follow inbuilt rules, that our lives are an expression of preordained patterns as predictable as the uncanny migration of salmon up the rivers at spawning time and the well-travelled flight paths of the returning swallows.

The literature of human development is crammed full with generalizations about the processes which we share, as humans of either sex or, specifically, as women. I searched it for patterns I could recognize, patterns which made sense of the plethora of experience I was uncovering. The idea which, for me, made the most sense was Jung's theory of individuation, which is why I have used it so persistently in this chapter.

As part of the theory, Jung had his own ideas about the differences between the male and female psyche. He believed that deep within the male is the inner female, or "anima," and likewise the inner male or "animus" is hidden within the outer persona of the female. For him, an important part of the individuation process was the uncovering of that hidden aspect, and that uncovering was—and still is—a key feature of Jungian analysis, the style of psychotherapy based on his work. I do believe that it is also a key feature in understanding the tasks of menopause, but not in exactly the form envisioned by Jung himself.

Perhaps, in Jung's day, it was a little easier to make generalizations about the psychological processes of development in men and women than it is now.

In his perception, as he looked around at his friends and relatives and patients, and inward into himself, it appeared that each human being was composed of both "male" and "female" qualities. That is to say, both sexes had the capacity for the so-called masculine behaviors and tendencies—competitiveness, strength, forcefulness, dynamism, and so on—and the so-called feminine ones—that is, receptivity, warmth, nurturing, gentleness, and so on. In a man's life, the masculine ones were more likely to be manifested, while the feminine ones were hidden within, and vice versa for the woman.

In the middle-class Swiss society which was Jung's environment, there would indeed have been evidence to suggest that these qualities belonged differentially to the two sexes in this way. Men would have usually been the breadwinners; women would probably have been at home rearing children. Men would generally have been expected to demonstrate their competence and aggressiveness by success in the outer world, such as the making of money and the building of business. Women would have been praised for their compliance and their gentle nurturance of their men and children. Such has been the way of many human societies.

In the West, we do not even have words for these two sets of qualities other than the words masculine and feminine. We seem to see a basic division into two sets of qualities, just as we see that there are two hemispheres of the brain, just as there is a bright, radiant sun and a gentle, reflective moon. Because we do not have words for those two categories, those two poles of being, the dynamic pole and the magnetic pole, and because we see some correlation between the two poles and the two sexes—in many species and in our own—we call them masculine and feminine. From this poverty of our language arises the idea that those qualities actually *are* masculine and feminine qualities. It is this sort of thing that I meant when I said in Chapter 1 that words can shape our thinking every bit as much as thinking shapes our words.

In the East, on the other hand, the ancient way of expressing the two poles is in the concept of yin and yang. Visually, yin and yang are depicted as the interdependent halves of the great whole, the whole which is all things, and which existed, undifferentiated, before all things, the Tao.

The yin/yang symbol, perfectly balanced, with each half containing the seed of the other, is a pictorial symbol with which many of us are familiar nowadays, but one whose full, rich meaning is not always completely understood.

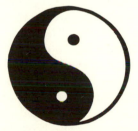

From that primordial wholeness of the Tao came the manifestation of the universe, brought into being by the interaction of the two great energies, yin and yang. Within the wholeness, all is maintained by that same interaction between the yin energy and the yang energy, and for anything to function properly, those two energies have to be in perfect balance and harmony.

Eastern medicine, for example, is based on that fundamental concept. For the human body to work perfectly, there has to be perfect balance between the yin and yang forces within that body. This, of course, includes the mind, since in Eastern thought there is no body/mind separation. As illustration, we can see in the macrobiotic diet, which has gained much popularity in the West in the past twenty years, a dividing of food into yin food and yang food. In simple terms, this is saying that if the body is out of balance by having too much of one or the other, we can simply adjust the proportions by eating the right food, and restore the yin/yang balance.

If we remove the connotations of biological gender from these two great forces that shape our world, we can see clearly that each of us has many ways of expressing yin energies and many ways of expressing yang energies. Certain functions we perform, as women, particularly the nurturing functions, demand large quantities of yin. However, if you have ever watched the actions of a mother—either human or other species—whose offspring are in danger, you would have seen the emergence of some very obvious yang activity. We have all heard stories of certain feats of superhuman strength which have been performed by women in such circumstances—physically lifting cars to release trapped babies and so on. In these, and in millions of smaller ways, women use their yang capabilities alongside the yin in everything they do.

The way in which they do it, however, is often subtly different from the way a man would do it, precisely because they *are* women. It is these differences which are now being explored, in our own times, as we penetrate more deeply into the mysteries to which Jung drew our attention.

Genia Pauli Hadden uses the symbolism of the human body to explain the differences, as she sees them, between the yin and yang energies of the two sexes. She points out that the so-called "male" energy has often been symbolized by the erect penis—that is, hard, thrusting, penetrating—whereas the receptive vagina has often seemed to typify the traditional passivity of the female.[3]

This imagery has been used in psychology in the past—for example, by Erik Erikson—whose research among children seemed to indicate that little boys typically built phallic structures in their games and little girls constructed hollow spaces.[4]

Hadden takes the physical metaphor much, much further.

She points out that the full reproductive apparatus of the mammal includes more than merely penis and vagina. The woman has a womb which is built of thick and sturdy muscle, the expulsive power of which is phenomenal. Likewise, below his active penis, the man wears the patient, passive testicles, the dark and nurturing seedbeds of his genes.

The special quality of yang power in a woman, explains Hadden, is like the special quality of power in the uterus. Unlike the random, blind thrusting of the penis, the womb's power is perfectly, exquisitely timed, and exactly sufficient for the occasion. Similarly, the yin energy of the male, symbolized by the testicles, is different again from the yin of the female. It has a quality of eternal patience and fidelity and it is that which we see in the most fully "developed" of men, a tenderness which is strong and unsentimental, a giving, but at exactly the right moments, and in the right quantities, not indiscriminately.

In addition to these highly appropriate energies, human beings often seem to display crude copies of each other which do not feel quite "right," especially to others. The weak, effeminate male is frequently disliked and lampooned, as is the bullying or nagging female, the one we call the harridan. A woman who tries to emulate men by adopting what she believes is a male way of doing things, in order to succeed in the world, may do so at a loss to herself and to others. However, in a world where the true feminine—that is, the full expression of both yin and yang in the female mode—has been undervalued, or not understood, that may have been the only way women could have made their voices heard. Now that our voices are being heard, we can begin to sing instead of to shout. To sing, not in the little, weak voices of the oppressed, but in the full-throated harmony of deep womanhood.

In the same way, men can now begin to discover their own deep maleness, with its true yin and its true yang, and as they do, the need for macho posturing may at last subside in our culture.

Jung, when he began his explorations into these realms, explained what he saw in terms of the animus and anima, the inner, contrasexual aspects. In the light of our deeper understanding of yin and yang, this may now seem simplistic. However, it did make sense of a phenomenon that Jung and others like him have recognized, and that is the change of emphasis which occurs at midlife.

Obviously, in a traditional society, if the outer male is to make a success of his life and survive as a breadwinner, his energies in the first part of adult life must be turned outward toward the world and to the workplace. His maleness befits him well for that role, for he has strong muscles, courage, determination, and all that it takes to carve his slice of the world. Similarly, the female's role during that time period is to tend the hearth and home and rear the children. Therefore, her nurturing feminine side will take easily to the task.

At midlife, when the children are grown and the fortunes of the family are secure, there is a tendency for each to turn back and begin to explore the hitherto-neglected aspects of self. The man may turn toward more nurturing ways of spending time—to farming or gardening, perhaps, or to service. He may do teaching or welfare of some kind. The Lions Club, Rotary, and suchlike are often full of older men who are performing selfless, nurturing tasks for the betterment of their communities. By the same token, midlife women have been flocking to the universities, thirsty for knowledge, or starting up businesses of their own with glee at their own boldness and successes. They have begun speaking with their own voices and demanding "me" time after half a lifetime of catering to the needs of their cared-for ones.

Jung saw this as men developing their neglected animas, or discovering the lost principle of "eros" within themselves, the yinlike principle of love and feelings, and women as finding and expressing the animus within and getting high on the "logos" principle of rationality, thinking, and knowledge.

In Jung's day, this all made perfect sense. Today, however, after many years of campaigning to end sex-role stereotyping, after many years of increasing opportunity for equality of the sexes in the work force, we find that the picture is far more confused. For example, I have been seeing women in my counseling practice who, in their midthirties, having risen high in their chosen professions after many years of devotion to outside activities, are now starting to long for babies. Others, through choice or economic necessity, have tried to combine both career and childrearing—the so-called "Supermom" syndrome—and wound up feeling that they have done neither really well or fully, and are burned out in the process of trying. Then there are men for whom the dominant male culture was so repugnant that they consciously tried to constellate their lives around different values and ended up feeling lost and alienated. They are sensitive and often feel that now they can no longer fit in their peer groups or relate to the pursuits and pastimes of those around them, and yet they long to relate deeply to other men. There are many permutations on these themes.

From this, I have drawn the conclusion that for many of today's women, there seem to be two crucial points of crisis.

The first, the well-known "midlife crisis," can come as early as the midthirties. This is the feeling that time is starting to run out and that the hitherto-neglected areas have to be attended to so that harmony and balance may be restored. At this time, it may be helpful to look at the balance of yin and yang in one's life and see whether there needs to be any correction of emphasis, any search for new ways to manifest these energies in the world.

The second crisis time is menopause. The new activities, eagerly embraced at thirty-five, with all the energy one had then, may now seem suddenly hard to maintain on the days of unexpected weariness or of the dreaded cotton-headed fuzziness. Menopause gives us permission to slow down. Not because we are "sick" or because we are in any way inadequate, inferior, or abnormal, but simply because the call has come. This is the sign, like the assembling of swallows on the wires, that a change of season is imminent. We must go inward and prepare; otherwise in our old age we shall have nothing to offer. The world will not need us forever to do what we are doing now. If what we are doing now is all that we know how to do, then eventually we shall become obsolete, rather than old and wise.

For some women, the two crisis points may run into one. A woman who has reared a large family, and whose youngest child is still a teenager when she draws near to fifty, or a woman who has been particularly involved in a fulfilling career, studded with a series of achievements, or especially a woman who has managed somehow to combine both of these—such a woman may experience one crisis point only. Of course, there may be many who do not even experience that for one reason or another. Since they will not be drawn to this book, I do not need to address them in detail here. After all, there is an old saying which reminds us, "If it works, don't fix it!"

I mention the notion of two crisis points here because there may well be women in their thirties who are experiencing puzzling changes in themselves and wondering if these could be something to do with early menopause. As a rule, it is unlikely that they are, although of course there are women who go through menopause unusually early. For younger women, the discussions of yin and yang energies, of the need to harmonize them, and of the need to put our own female signatures on our expressions of both yin and yang may still be highly relevant. So may the suggestions for deepening our understanding of ourselves through inner exploration. But if you are thirty-three, it may not yet be time to go deeply into a cocoon but time rather to seek out new directions, new pathways into the world before you start the homeward journey into the contemplative self.

That is not to say that we should not all engage in inner contemplation. Of course we should, and can at any age. It is merely that the natural emphasis in older age seems to be upon that inner journey, often to the exclusion of other concerns, and the input one gives to the world in older age is of a different quality somehow. It comes from a caring which is now more mellow and dispassionate, more gently accepting of anomalies and so-called "imperfections," more aware of the artificiality of all boundaries and polarities. More patient, perhaps.

We could possibly sum it up by saying that at thirty-five, at the peak of our energies, it may not be appropriate to put priority on the inner journey. The world needs our productivity and passion—our fertility, both biological and mental.

It needs our fiery energy to fight its fights and carry its crusades. The mellow wisdom of age has its own place in the scheme of things, and each comes forward at its time. Menopause, the time in the cocoon, is our rite of passage, our time out, in which we prepare ourselves to offer our services in that new way. It is the time when our menstrual blood, no longer shed, is turning alchemically to wisdom, and we, the vessels for that wisdom, are learning how our offerings may be poured.

In the next chapter we shall explore in more detail the special qualities of the postmenopausal woman. First, though, I would like you to withdraw again for a little while into reflection on your own experience and feelings.

* * *

Archeology and anthropology have revealed that in many cultures it has been a practice to equip the dead with supplies for some kind of posthumous journey to another world.

Into the tombs were put all that the people deemed necessary for that soul's sustenance. Food, crockery, clothing, symbolic and aesthetic objects, tools of many kinds, and so on.

In a way, menopause may be seen as a type of death. It is the death of who we have been, preceding the rebirth of who we shall become. The cocoon into which we crawl, in order for this transformation of ourselves to happen, is in many ways similar to the well-equipped tomb. I would like you to take a look at what you have provided for yourself in this time of metamorphosis.

Take a few moments to make an inventory.

1. Have you given yourself time and space? Are there periods of time which you can spend alone, in creative contemplation of your inner process? Places in which you have the privacy to weep or scream, move or dance, or simply be alone and quiet, uninterrupted by the work and routine of the outer world?

2. Have you given yourself freedom to explore? Have you let down the barriers which keep you from your inner expe-

rience? Have you assured yourself that it is O.K. to cry, to act crazy, to spend time doing nothing, to be "selfish?"

3. Have you taken hold of your right to explore and spend time alone? Have you been assertive in refusing any demands from other people which may interfere with or impose upon your necessary time in the cocoon? Have you renegotiated your outer commitments and shared routines so that time and space are available for your inner tasks?

4. Have you supplied yourself with the tools you need for the journey? Books, perhaps, to deepen your understanding. Journals to write in, crayons to write with, music to dance to or to inspire or calm you. Perhaps you may want to attend a workshop or some other group experience in order to share and deepen your own awareness. Maybe there are some special ritual objects you need to acquire. You may have to buy them. A beautiful candle perhaps, a statue, a bell, an incense burner, a special shawl or cushion. Or maybe you need to spend time in search of them, wandering among the tide pools or combing the forest floor, picking up shells at low tide or plucking a flower, finding a feather or a special stone. Whatever has special significance for you is a power thing. Power things are precious. You may be creating a medicine bundle for the emerging crone.

5. Have you begun to create your own forms? Once you have learned to be comfortable with private ritual, your creativity can emerge to enrich the outer rituals you share with others. Let your rituals flow from within, doing whatever feels just right in that moment. If it feels just right it will be right. It will be just what that moment needs.

6. Have you taken stock of your physical needs? Your body is changing and its needs may also be changing. Have you looked lately at your food, your intake of vitamins, your exercise regimen, your stress-management techniques? Are you getting enough sleep? If menopausal insomnia is bothering you, how are you compensating for this?

If you are not taking hormone replacements, have you investigated natural methods for aiding the physical process of menopause? Remember that you need regular, weight-bearing exercise in order to retard the bone-thinning process, and perhaps a review of your calcium intake as well.

Have you reviewed your clothing—its color, style, and texture? Are you letting yourself be guided by what feels good to wear, what feels right to you and looks right to your eyes, rather than what some outside authority or fashion fad dictates? Are you asking your body what it needs and learning to listen to its answers, rather than following the rules of some outside agency in matters of shape and diet, rest and sleep, health and healing, clothing and activity?

7. Have you taken the courage to reexamine everything? Your house and home, your lifestyle, your relationships and your work, your patterns of being in the world? Any or all of these may be up for reassessment now. Are you ready for the challenge? Your cocoon should be well equipped. Promise yourself that everything you need will be provided, in whatever way it can be achieved. Affirm it. This is your commitment to making menopause a significant event in your life. You will not regret the investment. It may cost nothing in dollars and cents, but it will probably have other costs. Whatever they are, I believe that they will be worth bearing.

7

WHO AM I BECOMING?

What is waiting for us? After menopause, the woman starts to turn into a crone. The sixth and final one of my themes of menopause is the theme of the crone.

Does the word "crone" make you wince a little? Or even shudder and mentally turn away? The word comes, after all, from the same rootstock as the word "carrion." The ancient word "croonie" was the word for an old ewe, a sheep that was soon to make a feast for crows. "Crone" is a plain, terrible, uncompromising word. Which is why we dwellers in a world of euphemisms and pastel curtains have a tendency to shrink from it. Yet in shrinking from it, and from all that it symbolizes, we are shrinking from our own power and potential.

I spoke, in an earlier chapter, of the Hindu Goddess Kali, a Goddess of fearsome visage, usually depicted with a string of skulls around her neck, dancing upon the body of her lover. Many travellers to the Indian subcontinent will have seen such images and been revolted or intrigued by them. Their credulity may be further strained by the discovery that the bloodthirsty Goddess is worshipped there with as much reverence and fervor as is given in other lands to the Virgin Mary, the beloved mother-saint of Christians. It seems bizarre. An unknown, alien strangeness, far from one's own experience.

The alienation, in fact, is within. In Western culture, we are so used to this inner alienation, this inner split, that we no longer notice its existence. Good and evil, right and wrong, light and dark, pleasure and pain, our entire vocabulary is the vocabulary of polarities, our whole experience the struggle of opposites, our life a constant series of battles between opposing forces. We inhabit a divided world. Our God represents the force of goodness, and his shadow, the Devil, is cast out of Heaven. Satan was the fallen angel. His banishment signifies, perhaps, our mythological remembrance of the original split in our cultural consciousness. Who knows?

The fact is that we, in the West, live with this chronic splitting. What is more, to follow the traditional God of the West is to perpetuate and deepen the split.

It seems there was a time, many, many centuries ago, when things were different. A time when life and death were seen to belong together, two parts of the same phenomenon. A time when human beings lived in balance with the rest of the natural world, living out their cycles with the seasons and the moons and all the other circular patterns of coming and going, rising and falling. Women gave birth, as women always have. And in the minds of those ancient peoples, all life began with the female. The fecund mother was the origin of all things. In the haunting words of Merlin Stone, "In the beginning, people prayed to the Creatress of Life, the Mistress of Heaven. At the very dawn of religion, God was a woman. Do you remember?"[1]

Maybe it was so. Stone's research, taking us back along the highways of history to uncover the archeological evidence for widespread worship of the Goddess, is certainly persuasive. Certainly I believe it. But whether you believe it or not is up to you. Perhaps it does not really matter what happened back in history. It does not matter whether those women who were our ancient ancestors held the power in their society and worshipped a female God, or whether they did not. The real point is that these archetypal forms yield up a rich and vivid symbolism for the women of today, bringing them a new power and understanding. Even if the Goddess were purely a fantasy, her power would still be the same. As one feminist writer explains it,

A remembered fact and an invented fantasy have identical
psychological value. The matriarchies, i.e. the times when no
woman was the slave of any man, create visions of the pride
and power women are working to have in their present lives.
Thus matriarchies are functioning in modern covens and in
modern witches' dreams whether or not societies ruled by females ever existed in past history.[2]

The message which we can gain from the stories and rituals
of the Goddess is that the true world is not split. Man and
Nature are not separate. If the rainforest dies we all die. Birth
and death are not separate. They are two aspects of the same
process. God and the Devil are not separate. They are two
sides of the same coin.

Whenever we try to deny or ignore one side of any of our
pairs of opposites, we only empower it. Whenever one strives
to be kind, without acknowledging one's ability to be cruel,
to profess love without tapping one's capacity to hate, to seek
happiness and run away from pain, one is like a handcuffed
person trying to move one hand. It is only when we see our
pairs for what they are, two-sided coins whose sides cannot
be separated and who depend upon each other for existence,
that we can begin to understand.

As Jungian psychology maintains, we cannot find the self
until we have accepted the shadow. In order to reach our full
potential as human beings, we must accept ourselves in all
our aspects, our so-called vices along with our so-called vir-
tues. There is no happiness without sadness, for each must
exist in order to define the other. There are no peaks without
valleys. The only alternative is a flat plain, and even the words
"flat plain" would cease to exist if there were no peaks or
valleys, since all the world would be a flat plain and therefore
would not need defining. Without death, there can be no life.
Without the crone, no other woman can be born.

The path to this type of deep understanding is not through
intellect as much as through experience. That is the beauty
of the Goddess. She, in all her guises, leads us to understanding. Unlike the distant God who, no matter how close we may
come to him, remains always separate from ourselves, the

Goddess is us, and we are her. The Goddess, like us, is a
woman.

Kali, the destroyer, the remorseless taker of life, is but the
flip side of Kali the creator, mother of all things. Like the earth
itself, all things come from her, all things return to her. There
is no escape from the endless cycle of birth and death. It
matters little whether the icon depicts the mother-god with
blood dripping from her teeth, in an orgy of destruction, or
in a gown of blue with the infant in her arms. Mary, queen
of heaven, and Kali the terrible Goddess are one and the same.
So is Demeter, with her sheaves of corn, and her daughter
Persephone, and all the other Goddesses of Greece. So is the
Spider-Woman in her lair and Pele in her fiery furnace. All
are aspects of the one Goddess. All the aspects of the Goddess
live within us, within every woman. They may live only as
potential, as a possibility, a choice, a yet-to-be-explored option. Yet in some form, they are all there.

Could you kill? At some level we all kill. Whether it is the
killing of another human being—in war, in defense, in anger,
in euthanasia—or the purchase of a frozen chicken or the
slicing of a turnip for the family's soup, we all kill. At some
level, we destroy life daily, or cause it to be destroyed. Life
lives on life, and death daily serves the living. That is the
nature of life on earth. Deep down, every woman knows that.

Could you give birth? A baby, a project, an idea, or the
rebirth of self in a new unfolding of consciousness. Planting
a seed, drawing up a contract, building a house. We all give
birth. The very cells of our bodies renew themselves over and
over again, dividing, multiplying, birthing. Life is constant,
irrepressible birth. That, too, is the natural order of things.

All of life is a constant interplay, a dance of birthing and
dying. Within you, right now, cells are dying, cells are birthing. Within you there is Mary, and there is Kali, and within
you all the others live, too, each in her own way.

Jean Shinoda Bolen speaks of the "Goddesses in Everywoman," the rising and falling of the different Goddess aspects in each woman's life, the recognizable patternings to
which the Greeks gave women's names—Athena, Artemis,
Hestia, and all the rest.[3]

In our differing personalities and the varied experiences of our lives, we may each manifest the various qualities and tendencies of the Goddesses in a host of different ways and different blends. Athena the intellectual, voluptuous Aphrodite, untamed Artemis, jealous Hera, we can be one of them or some, or all of them in turn, across a lifetime. Likewise, we may breathe with Pele's volcanic fire at one moment and heal with the gentle compassion of Kwan Yin at the next.

The point is that no matter what aspect of the Goddess we are manifesting, we embody her rather than speak to her as "other," the way, as children, we were taught to speak to our God or his representatives.

I did not always know this. At some deep level, it was something I had searched for, yet I did not know what it was that I was seeking.

My mind goes back to fifteen-year-old me. The gauche, uncertain child, learning to live in a body that was becoming woman. Struggling with new feelings, with mysterious and unspoken passions, and above all with deep, existential doubts, I spent a long time pondering on the meaning of things and the nature of God.

I remember a certain summer day, a Sunday. I had plucked up courage to announce that I was not going to church. This was an unwelcome announcement which earned me a considerable amount of disapproval. Despite it all, I held out, surly in my insistence on making my choice. Church time came and I was alone, in new, dearly won freedom which carried a tinge of guilt for my defiance, and for my surliness. I went outside, into the morning sunshine.

The church was nearby, across a meadow. I remember so vividly sitting in the warm grass, amongst the gentle hum and buzz of bees and other insects, the sun blessing me. Birds twittered. The leaves on the trees rustled. The air was scented with summer.

From the church I could just dimly hear the dull drone of a hymn. I looked across in pity at the squat, stone building, hunched in its graveyard. I knew it would be cold in there. I knew the people would be dutifully turning the pages of their prayer books, locked into what I saw as dull and lifeless rituals, their minds elsewhere, their hearts unopened and their eyes unseeing.

Maybe I was wrong. How could I, a fifteen-year-old girl, know what was happening inside the minds and bodies of those men and women? Maybe I was wrong. But to me, under the blue sky, the blessings were raining down in the meadow, and all of Nature was laughing at the foolishness of human beings who seek their God inside stone walls on a summer's day. I felt sacredness all around me. Whatever God was, God was there, with me.

Since I had always been taught that God was male and God was "other," I simply decided that I had figured out where he liked to spend his time. Indeed, I felt smug. For I knew where to find him, and had his whole attention, while all those stupid people were huddled in the church singing hymns. Hymns which both God and I knew were exceedingly boring. We giggled together that day, my God and I, united in our truancy.

The feeling never left me. Even in the darkest moments, there was always the sense of an unseen companion beside me. There was always the cozy knowledge of a private, privileged relationship with God—or at least with one of his representatives—which was outside the accepted forms and rituals of society.

But still my God was "other." Near or far, in whatever form, there was always the separation. Someone walked with me but he was not me and I was not him.

When I first began to read about the rediscovery of the ancient Goddess religions which existed for millenia before the coming of the patriarchal, male God, I was excited. When I read of the deliberate, savage campaigns to wipe out those religions and the matrilineal cultures which went with them and to replace them with the God of the Hebrews, I felt grief and outrage. Even more outrage when I read about the many millions of women who were persecuted and swept away to oblivion in a great, attacking, male campaign that was at least twice as big as the Holocaust of our own century and just as cruel and irrational, the campaign against witchcraft, carried out in the name of Christianity.

At first, the outrage was disabling. Then, as time went on, I worked my way through it to a deeper understanding. I began to realize that man's fear of death had led him, over the centuries of human history, to try to find ways to overcome it, to make himself immortal and invincible. In the process, there was a rejection of all that the Goddess stood for. As Barbara Walker puts it, "The life given by Mother was always cyclic, never eternal. For some men it was never enough. They wanted a life everlasting."[4] Man's craving to overcome death, to conquer Nature and make the universe serve him, in the name of a patriarchal God, caused him to turn against woman, that ever-present symbol of cyclicity and death. Yet he needed her, for she was also life. So he learned to tame and oppress her. He split her. He set upon his pedestal of adoration those aspects which he loved—her nubile beauty and her nurturing motherhood—and set about trying to stamp out the death-dark aspects of her which he found so fearsome, those aspects which reminded him of his mortality and of the futility of his quest to overcome death and finitude. Woman, as witch, became the enemy to be routed, the weed to be uprooted wherever it grew.

As women we embody cyclicity. We wax and wane, ovulate and menstruate, month after month for around forty years. The very processes of our bodies serve to remind us, and the men who share our world, that life itself is cyclic. It begins in the darkness before birth and it returns to the same darkness after death. Our female lives begin in smooth, straight, nonfertile bodies, and bud into nubile virginity. We flower as women, nurture new life, and then die back as wise crones, sinewy with a lifetime's wisdom, hinting at death.

Christianity took two phases of the cycle and exalted them as one denatured Goddess. Mary, queen of heaven, was virgin and mother in one. She was worshipped on her pedestal. But the crone, the third member of the holy trinity, was banished. She became the witch who was feared and burned. All the ugliness, the fear of death, was projected onto her. The further she was banished, the more mischief she made, like the witch of the fairy tale who did not get invited to the party. The more we disown our shadow—the disliked parts of ourselves that

we cannot accept or acknowledge—the more mischief it
makes in our lives. The more we disown it, the more we project
it onto others and then damn them with our judgments. The
Inquisition was a mass projection. Women bore the brunt of
it then and have lived with the wounds of it ever since, as any
feminist text will testify.

In splitting and suppressing female power, man only served
to split and suppress his own true nature and deny his own
potential. As Neumann puts it,

> [The] male principle of consciousness which desires perma-
> nence and not change, eternity and not transformation, law
> and not creative spontaneity, "discriminates" against the
> Great Goddess and turns her into a demon.
>
> But in so doing, the male consciousness totally overlooks the
> hidden, spiritual aspect of the feminine principle, which
> through spiritual transformation exalts earthly man to a higher
> meaning.[5]

Whatever holds true for individuals is in some way reflected
in the whole. Thus the suppression of the "feminine principle"
of which Neumann speaks is the root cause of much that
troubles us today on a worldwide scale. There are splits at a
worldwide level. Which is only to be expected since, in his
words, "the Great Mother not only spins human life but also
the fate of the world, its darkness as well as its light."[6]

However, we must start where we are. If we are to heal the
wounds of the past and begin to heal the dangerous and potentially fatal splits in today's world—between race and race,
men and women, humanity and Nature—then we must begin
by healing the inner splits. Only when the splits within us are
healed can we hope to heal the outer ones. Some of our work,
inside the cocoon, is to search for those inner splits and to
reclaim the disowned parts of our own nature. We can take
time, for instance, to notice the things about other people that
deeply bother us and recognize them as being, in fact, projected parts of our own selves. This is humbling, healing work.

Menopause is a signal that we are entering crone territory.
Wonderful as it may have been to have sat on that pedestal

as virgin and as mother—those two aspects of womanhood that not only the Christian religion but also our popular culture loves to love—now the pedestal has to be vacated. Society is still having great difficulty with the crone. No pedestal yet for her. The trouble is, society will not be able to honor her out there until we ourselves can honor her within us. Inasmuch as we have allowed our own taming process to take place, now we must reclaim our inner wildness.

So why do we flinch from her? Why do we look askance at Kali? I think it is because we know that the time for splitting has ended. We are about to become old. We can no longer postpone the time when the image of the old woman and the face in the mirror start to fuse. Old age and death must be faced now.

> Menopause is a time for confronting death while there is still time to live. It is a true initiation, a doorway through death to a new phase of life. Fear of natural menopause, fear of the Crone, translates also into dread of death. Through bodily experiences of yang-femininity, in both menstruation and menopause, women (and men who relate sensitively to them) have opportunities to encounter the dark death side of the Divine.[7]

Kali epitomizes the "dark death side of the Divine." I knew that one of my main menopausal tasks was to come to terms with Kali. The symbolism inherent in that Kali image was one of the things I needed in order to negotiate my way through this stage of my life. But I was fearful.

So often, for me, change begins with the intellect and then seeps into the feelings and then finally is acknowledged at a bodily, cellular level. That was how it was with Kali. I saw her, as I had always seen my Gods, as "other." I knew, because I had been immersed in the study of menopause, that somehow I had to come to an intimate relationship with this old, dark creature, but I was terrified. I wrote about it and drew pictures, but the fear remained. Then one evening, as I took a shower before bedtime, a strange thing happened. I looked up and saw the vision of a hand, holding the edge of the shower curtain. It was an old and wrinkled hand, dry like leather,

and very dark. I knew it was Kali's hand. I knew that I was
not yet ready to look her in the face but that the process of
acceptance had begun. I was able to look at her hand and
remain calm. I knew, also, that Kali, in her compassion, had
edged herself in gently, so that I could open to her. This
thoughtfulness touched me. As I looked at the hand, a feeling
of love swept over me. I began to sing a quiet hymn to Kali.
I was beginning to let her in.

From that time, the fear of aging left me. Concern over my
drying skin and aging body left me. There was a peacefulness
in place of it, a peacefulness which has remained.

By the time I was ready to look Kali in the face, I knew that
it would not happen anywhere else but in the mirror. Somehow, somewhere in the last few years an important shift has
happened. I now know that the Goddess, unlike the God of
my childhood, is not out there to be worshipped. She is in
here to be experienced. My own life is a manifestation of her.

Feminist theologian Nelle Morton describes a plane journey
she took in 1976 in which she became very frightened in a
storm and, rather than calling upon God the Father to protect
her, decided to invoke the Goddess instead. Almost immediately, an unseen presence came to her side and gave her in-
structions for dealing with the fear in her body, taking her
from panic to a sense of joy and freedom, leaving her strong
and unafraid. "I began to feel such power within, as if she
had given me myself. She had called up my own energy."

When Nelle opened her eyes, there was no one there to
thank. "A new thing I recognized immediately: the Goddess
works herself out of business. She doesn't hang around to
receive thanks. It appears to be thanks enough for her than
another woman has come into her own."[8]

There is an exultation in me now which was never there in
all the earlier years of my life. It is an inner joy that comes
from knowing the Goddess and feeling her within me, breathing my breath, living my life through me, empowering me.

It could never have been like that with a male God. How
could it have been? How could a male God live in a woman's
body? I could love a male God and respect him, walk with
him, turn to him for advice, worship him even, but I could

not feel that he was me. Although I never lost the sense of having a personal, unseen male companion who walked with me, my idea of God in adulthood became abstract and metaphysical. If ever I was asked to define God, I spoke in vague, mystical concepts. Directly experienced, God was to me an all-pervading sense of sacredness, a unity, a special something at the center of creation, which had no name or gender. This experience was only available at certain times, however, such as in deep meditation, or at peak moments. At other times, I felt out of touch with it, lost, with only the memory of those experiences to sustain me. In contrast, the Goddess feeling is with me almost all the time now. This has been the gift of my menopause.

I have been the virgin and the mother. Now I am becoming the crone. The word no longer makes me flinch. On the contrary, it thrills me. It is a power word. A word of fullness and completion. There is a richness in it which I never dreamed of a few years ago.

There is also a new lightness. A new, economical lightness which gives the same sense of satisfaction as travelling with a very light backpack.

Maybe it is because my body no longer becomes bloated and heavy; my breasts are light and soft instead of full and fleshy. Maybe it is because I feel so much more freedom to be whatever I want to be in the moment instead of having to maintain a certain sort of image. In a way, it is like regaining the freedom of childhood while retaining the wisdom of a life's experience. Whatever it is, I love this emerging lightness.

Sometimes I have the fantasy that as I become an old woman I shall get lighter and lighter, like a leaf. When it is time to die, I shall be so light that I can easily be lifted, like a child, onto my dying-place and my spirit will float effortlessly from this body, like smoke on the breeze.

Yet there is still a deep caring and commitment. There is still fire inside me, but the years have matured it into the clear heat of glowing coals rather than the leaping flames of impassioned youth.

Other women speak, too, of this lightness. One drew a picture of herself and her family. The figures of her husband and children were clustered together and heavily drawn but she herself, penciled in light, almost impressionistic strokes, was moving forward, away from them, though still part of their group. Her figure was surrounded by radiant light. The picture gave a strong sense of lightness and light-heartedness, while retaining the impression of deep caring. Describing her picture, she simply said, "I am now free to experience the world in a new, 'light' way."

Carmel is divorced and lives alone. She is forty-eight, and her menopause process is only just beginning, yet she is already feeling intimations of the new lightness in herself. For her, it is experienced as an increasing simplicity in her days and in all her activities, even though she follows a busy, active lifestyle. Life seems more spiritual, she says, yet it is a spirituality which is now immanent in ordinary, everday things. In her words:

> The spiritual and other dimensions are finally merging. For example, I note that I can watch my granddaughter play and not feel that I "ought" to be doing something more important. ...I've also been re-reading Krishnamurti and he emphasizes this unity of the spiritual and everyday reality so this has helped me to confirm this. I'm more willing to just be with people and not consider that it is frivolous.

The lightness, the simplicity, these are aspects of the crone that were a surprise to me, presumably because until now I had always looked at the crone from the outside. Now I am starting to feel her from the inside.

Do you remember the African woman we met in Chapter 1, whose menopausal status brought her an immunity from danger because it emptied her life of any meaningful role in the tribe? One now wonders whether she, too, experienced her new definition—of nonperson—as a lightness. Maybe she did. Maybe it was the best time of her life. Who knows?

I suspect, however, that freedom without involvement brings only a sense of alienation. I am sure, too, that our society's attitudes toward old age create more alienation than they do a light and joyous freedom.

Far from being valued as a repository of wisdom or as a ceremonial leader, in modern Western society the crone is often relegated to the role of "little old lady." As such she is at best ignored or patronized and at worst, beaten.

A few years ago Pat Moore, a thirty-two-year-old industrial designer, hatched the idea of disguising herself as an eighty-five-year-old woman in order to find out more about society's elderly. Her aim was to learn how she could accommodate her product designs more appropriately to the needs of older people. Pat walked the streets of New York for three years, off and on, fascinated and horrified by what she was discovering. Her experiment revealed a world in which the elderly, particularly women, were subject to contempt, ridicule, and even physical abuse. It was a profoundly shocking revelation.[9]

Our modern society, in little more than a century, has turned on its head the natural developmental sequence which had prevailed for all of human history. This was a sequence in which the elders of society, having lived the major part of their lives in active interaction with their environment, were seen as

> the transmitters of tradition, the guardians of ancestral values and the providers of continuity. They were awarded such titles as sage, patriarch, seer, and venerable counselor and were consulted as advisors and sometimes as prophets, since long-range memories make prediction, founded on experience, trustworthy. Their life-histories provided the warp on which the lively threads of the ongoing community were in the process of being woven.[10]

What a wonderful image of involvement and wholeness. Sadly, things have changed. Nowadays, in this information age, where even the latest computer is outdated in a year and knowledge is increasing at an exponential rate, it is the young who make the predictions. The grandchild knows more than the father and twice as much as the grandfather. More, that is, of the knowledge the world seems to value. What that knowledgeable child does not have, of course, is wisdom. Which may be why the age of technology is bringing the life-forms on our planet to a survival crisis.

Somehow, we must rediscover wisdom. The crone has wisdom sorely needed in the world, but as little old lady, bent in alienation and lost in feeble retirement, vacuously ticking off her days in front of a TV, she has lost the power to deliver it. She has bought the empty products of a technological, materialistic world and absorbed the values of a sexist, ageist culture, and she has lost her meaning.

If this is the fate of the crone, little wonder that we flinch from it. Bad enough that we should have to endure the loss of all that which gave us recognition—the "good looks," the sexual desirability, the ability to bear children—but menopause also forces us to contemplate our imminent entry into a no-woman's-land of uselessness and nonpersonhood.

As Simone de Beauvoir once put it:

> From the day a woman consents to growing old, her situation changes. Up to that time she was still a young woman, intent on struggling against a misfortune that was mysteriously disfiguring and deforming her; now she becomes a different being, unsexed but complete: an old woman. It may be considered that the crisis of her "dangerous age" has been passed. But it should not be supposed that henceforth her life will be an easy one. When she has given up the struggle against the fatality of time, another combat begins: she must maintain a place on earth.[11]

Here we have the menopausal women in a state of dread. If the models she sees before her are the women who have meekly succumbed to being little old ladies with no meaning in their lives and no status in their human groupings, what is there to inspire her to cross that bridge of menopause with trumpets blaring and flags flying?

Such a woman "has and is a problem. She is in limbo, or at least she is in transition. The models for womanhood presented by her mother and grandmother are no longer useful. She has to fumble through and make her own paths, much of the way by trial and error."[12]

Some of us are more fortunate than others in that we do have positive role models to follow. In every age, no matter

how persecuted, the crone has always been visible somewhere, manifesting in women of strength, power, and wisdom.
Sometimes, the crone reveals herself in a new fearlessness, a
new unconcern with stuffy morality, a new bawdiness that
raises eyebrows. The crone can be outrageous and enjoy every
moment of her outrageousness. She can be an iconoclast, up-
ending the carefully set tables of convention with a cackle,
daring us to follow the pointing of her finger, to reexamine
habit, to awaken to new understandings.

Jennifer, a counselor whose clientele are mostly lesbian
women, finds that menopause is often the stage of life when
women are at last able to "come out" as lesbians after a
lifetime of denial and masquerade. With this emergence
comes a new, fresh honesty and forthrightness that can shock
friends and relatives, and also a revitalized sexuality and a
surge of libido. Certainly a very different scenario from the
standard one proposed by so many books on menopause.

While the virgin is powerful but untouchable and the
mother has her arms full with nurturing tasks, the crone is
wild and free. She can relate at will or not relate at all. In
this sense she, too, is virgin, in the true meaning of the word—
that is, she is unpossessed by any man. She is her own woman.
As virgin again, she joins hands with the young virgin of the
trinity, thus completing the circle.

The crone has the freedom to please herself. She can stand
aloof or roll up her sleeves and join in. She has the keys to
all doors. In order to open them, however, she has to know
her power.

The power of the crone is a female power, which is the power
to give birth, to transform, to shift shapes, to create. It is not
the "power over" of the male world, the bossiness of hierar-
chies or the control of men and women by a dictator. This
female power, which is the secret of the crone, is what
Adrienne Rich calls "the truly significant and essential
power."[13] It is a power which can heal. There is a lot of healing
needed in the world at this point in history. I believe that the
things which have gone wrong in the world are mostly trace-
able to the excesses of male-type power. By this, I do not mean

the sins or mistakes of individuals of either gender, but the imbalances which have come as part of the process of social evolution.

The environmental crisis, for example, has come about because man, backed by his religious convictions, believed that he had power over Nature and a mandate to "subdue" her. The crisis of inequality, of Third World poverty, has come about because of the greedy seeking for the same kind of power, the power over people, resources, and money. If ever there were the right time for the resurgence of true female power and wisdom it is now. It may be the last and only chance we have to save our lopsided world. Not by women becoming pseudo-men and fighting their way to the tops of corporate trees in order to prove that they are "as good as men," but by women asserting their true female power, balancing their inner yin and yang and, one by one, speaking the truth of who they are and what they believe in.

"When women begin to feel confident and to express the values of their own way of being, then they will enable the healing of the masculine."[14]

The answer does not lie in blaming men. It lies in taking powerful action. The patriarchal society only survives because women have complacently agreed to become its infrastructure and support its ways and its values. Imagine a world where no woman ever bought a product unless she had absolute proof that in its making no creature, either human or animal, had suffered or been exploited and no pollution had been caused; she would require proof that no sexism, ageism, or racism, however subtle, had been employed in its advertising, that no undue profit had been wrung from its sale, and that no unethical investment or practice was followed by its producers. She would insist that its packaging be minimal and recyclable.

Imagine a world where no woman would relate in any way to men whose attitudes were sexist, ageist, racist, polluting, or exploitative, even fathers, husbands, brothers, and sons. Remember the story of Lysistrata? When women do use their power, it works. It is the crone within each of us that dares to use power in this way.

Imagine a modern Western country in which, one morning, every woman in the land decided that her work hours should henceforth fit her needs and rhythms, rather than the other way around. What chaos would ensue! Eventually, though, the workplace may begin to change to accommodate the needs of women, whether it be for time and space to breast-feed, rearranged schedules for PMS, or time out for an episode of menopausal "fuzzy-brain."

The first step to using our power is to feel it. The only way to feel it is to allow ourselves fully to feel all of our female experience. This means the turbulence of adolescence and the natural rhythms of menstruation. It means the full expression of our sexuality in whatever form we choose to manifest it. If we desire it, it includes pregnancy, childbirth, and lactation. It also means all the feelings and events of menopause. It includes all the phases and stages of our life, the changing, shifting influences of the Goddesses within us and the personal, unique experience of being this particular woman in this particular body at this particular moment in history.

Our power, at menopause, is shifting within us. From henceforth it will manifest differently in the world. Eventually, when the process is complete, each of us will be a crone, and crone power is a formidable force. Since it is an integral part of the whole, it is of course within us at any age, as potential, but it is after menopause that crone power is most strongly embodied, if we can allow it to come through us.

Elissa Melamed, whose words on aging I quoted in the previous chapter, believes that this power is not being taken up because women have bought the values and images of the patriarchal culture. After interviewing over 200 women in seven countries, she sees the youth fixation and women's consequent inability to take hold of their authority as they age as contributing factors to the lopsidedness of the current political structure of the planet. Older women, she says, "are currently our most under-utilized natural resource."[15]

If we take the option of being little old ladies, passive and unstimulated by life, filling our time with mind-numbing pastimes, our power will be lost to us and our own wisdom will decay inside us long before we die. A woman who shuffles into an old age characterized by what one writer called a "dubious uroboric drowsing as a quasi-patient"[16] has no function other than to wait for the end, her waiting at best enlivened by TV or occupational therapy in place of the missing sense of meaning.

Simone de Beauvoir, writing in the days before she herself became old, wrote an acerbic catalogue of the roles played out by older women in her society.[17] She saw women who had lived only for their children now dominating their children's lives in ever-more desperate and futile attempts to maintain the control which was the only form of power they knew. She saw women whose lives had failed to fulfill them striving to shape their children and proteges to fit their own needs for vicarious success.

These were women who clung to their earlier roles when the roles had through time become obsolete. They were unable to let go of the roles or of the people who had shared in the casting. "Nothing is rarer," said de Beauvoir, "than the mother who sincerely respects the human person in her child, who recognizes his liberty even in failure."[18]

Not only are women often unable to free their children from the outlived forms of the past, they may also attempt to absorb their grandchildren into the same forms. The only life they know is the old one.

De Beauvoir saw women whose days were made of emptiness filling their time with idle gossip, pointless tasks, and artificially manufactured meaning. These patterns of living are still with us. I see them daily in my counseling practice. Women who cannot let go of their children, who squabble over their grandchildren, who cling to the old life. Women who expect their families to create meaning for them long after those families have grown up and left.

That is not to say, of course, that our families cannot continue to be a source of pride and pleasure, of rich relating and deep fulfillment. There is an ineffable joy in watching one's offspring grow and develop, and that joy does not diminish when they reach adulthood. It extends to our grandchildren or to the students of our students and to all those whose lives we have touched and nourished with gifts of self. But we must simply watch, not attempt to control.

It is all too easy to get caught up in issues of achievement and accomplishment, to feel proud at graduations, to want the lives of those we love to be filled with happiness and glory. We must also remember that to struggle and to learn, to suffer and to come through pain are also the privileges of being human. One of the principal tasks of parenting is learning to hand over to our children the responsibility to search for their own opportunities. Much as it hurts to watch, we can feel proud when they stumble, proud when they do their own falling, in their own way, and learn their own ways of picking themselves up again. Like pots in the kiln, they will be stronger for the baking. This holds as true for our proteges, our clients, our students, or any others whom we have nurtured along the way as it does for the children we have physically borne, adopted, or fostered. It holds true, too, for all our children, in any degree of impairment. Even a profoundly retarded child can reach out for autonomy in tiny ways. I taught Susan to flush the toilet. It took many weeks of patient repetition, but in the end she learned, and I was proud. She had achieved that tiny piece of autonomy and I could take one small step back.

I am remembering the poignant scene at the airport when my elder daughter first took a plane alone to Europe. Eighteen years old, with big, eager eyes and shining hair, she looked so vulnerable standing there with her new backpack and a slight tremble in the hands that reached out for the boarding pass. We had talked for months about her flying, like a young bird, from the nest-home, and about my tendency to twitter anxiously and doubt the strength of those young wings. She was scared and excited by turns, flip-flopping from one state to the other in the same day. As the time drew nearer, she flip-flopped several times an hour, and by the day itself she was down to every few seconds. "I'm so excited/I'm so scared!" After a final hug, she walked through the barriers, a thin slip of humanity, holding herself carefully, alone now, eyes wet. She turned, just before she moved out of sight, and with her

hands by her sides made little wing-flapping motions, grinning
an uncertain grin at me through the tears. Then she was gone.

Some time later, from Paris, came a beautiful postcard. It
showed an open hand, and from the hand flew a white bird.
No words. On the back she had written, "Mommy, you set me
free, and now I am free and flying. I can do anything. Nothing
is beyond me. Here's to happiness, and a friendship that will
never die."

I put the card in my purse. Next day, I told the story in one
of my groups and showed the card to some of the women. One
woman began to cry. Her young son had been refusing to go
to school. She realized that it was her pain, her clinging, that
was holding him, and she began to release it.

This is how, as women, we can heal each other. As we share
our stories, our deep feelings, the healing spreads; the wisdom
that is within all of us is channeled to where it is needed, like
irrigation water.

Crones have inner reservoirs of that wisdom, and their task
is to channel it into the world in whatever way seems necessary, whether large or small.

I am remembering my grandmother. Her wisdom came in
funny little sayings that I treasure to this day. Quaint little
Victorian adages, but they guide me still. *"Comparisons are
odious." "Clean the corners and the middle will look after itself."
"Plenty more pebbles on the beach." "Pride must pinch."* They
come tumbling out of memory when I recall her voice with
its gentle, Devonshire accent, her plump, cuddly figure, the
smell of her baking and the feel of her lap. The archetypal
grandmother we all like to remember. I was lucky to have
one of those. Perhaps that is how my grandchildren will remember me, for certainly she is a strong model, a Demeter
figure I have enjoyed emulating. But I know that in some way
there will be more added, when my turn comes. For my grandmother was a passive daughter of the patriarchy who never
questioned the values of her society and her church. She was
inward-looking, toward her family, neither knowing nor caring much for the machinations of the wider world. The crone
I am becoming will be different. She is waspier, saltier, more
hard-edged. She will have a wider territory perhaps, more

trees to mark with her wisdom-scent. Not better, just different.

As personal grandmother, in relationship with my own children's children, I hope I can be as de Beauvoir suggests:

> Recognizing neither rights nor responsibilities, she loves them in pure generosity; she does not indulge in narcissistic dreams through them, she demands nothing of them, she does not sacrifice to them a future she is never to see. What she loves is simply the little beings of flesh and blood who are present here and now.[19]

I also know that in my life there will always be a wider dimension beyond the family. For the sort of crone which I am becoming, this is imperative.

Crones like me have to move back out into the world, giving whatever we feel like giving, doing whatever we feel like doing, laughing at the absurdity of existence. We must let life move through us, let its rhythms touch us, lend our wisdom in whatever ways it is called out from us.

Even if we do not have models to guide us, we can create them. Deep in the collective unconscious of all womankind are the myths and secrets of the witch and the midwife, the powerful archetypal patterns of the Goddess. We can channel them out into the world, for healing, for renewal, or even just for fun. We can play our full parts in this beautiful melodrama of life, until we die.

A Meditation

You may like to try this simple routine for bringing into your body the physical experience of openness and power. It need take only a few minutes.

First, take off your shoes. Now, take some big, deep breaths, expelling the air with a big HA!

Next, spend a little time just stretching and shaking your arms, hands, feet, legs, and so on, until your whole body begins to feel loose, warm, and relaxed. You will then be ready to do the meditation.

Stand with your feet approximately shoulder-width apart. Your knees should be very slightly bent, or at least "unlocked," and your spine should be comfortably straight. Let your arms hang loosely by your sides, with your hands open.

Keep your eyes open, lightly resting at some point in the middle distance, but unfocused and soft.

Let your body relax. Become aware of your breathing. Do not alter it; simply become aware of it. Every time you breathe out, feel yourself relax. Let your mind go quiet, resting.

As you breathe, become aware of the feeling of your feet, planted squarely on the ground. Feel them there, firm and solid. Feel the openness of your body as you stand there, strong and steady, your arms by your sides.

Feel the surges of energy coming up from the ground, through the soles of your feet, up your legs, into your belly. Feel the power as it builds up within you. Feel your strength.

After a few minutes, shake our your arms and legs again and resume your normal activities with a renewed feeling of vigor and centeredness.

Some women find it quite strange to stand in this "open" way. Many of us have been taught to arrange our bodies in "ladylike" patterns and tend to keep our arms in front of us, our feet together, and, when we are sitting, our legs or feet crossed. You may care to observe yourself and to notice, in your daily activities, how much time you spend with your body guarded and arranged in these well-learned ways. You could experiment with doing it differently and see how it feels. I have a theory that the more open and relaxed our bodies are in their environment, the more open our hearts are to the world and the more available our power is to be used.

8

LIVING THE MENOPAUSE

Menopause, as we have been speaking of it throughout this book, is not simply a biological process. It is a phase of each woman's life. It may be short or long, complicated or simple, dramatic or subtle, problematical or easy. For each woman, it will be slightly different, with different components, a unique flavor. Just as each of us has her unique scent, her unique set of fingerprints, each of us has her way of experiencing menopause and living it. Let us converse, as women all over the world have talked together since the beginning of speech. That is how we learn and grow. Tell me about your menopause.

How are you living it? How is it for you? Has it barely begun or is it well under way? Maybe it is ending, or ended.

A little while ago, my best friend, who is some years younger than me, read part of an early draft of this book. Physiologically, no menopausal symptoms had appeared in her life, and yet she sensed changes in herself, changes with which she had been quietly struggling for some time, trying to make sense of them. She had felt anxious, uncertain, puzzled. The woman who was her seemed to be changing in subtle ways she could not easily define. Her thinking was becoming different. More hazy, less crisp and logical. After she read the pages and we had talked, she began to realize that she is, in fact, engaged in the beginning of a perfectly natural process.

Her menopause is beginning. She is entering the world of cotton-head and fuzzy-brain, of weary days and teary days, of zestful times and new music to which she needs to dance. She is finding herself on a journey with no clear destination— a road with sudden, concealed turnings and perhaps more than a few potholes. My friend is entering a rite of passage. She will emerge one day from the other end and she will have started to become a crone.

Has your process begun? How did it begin? Maybe, like many women, the first thing to come to your notice was physical change. A period that was lighter than usual, or did not arrive, an unaccustomed feeling of heat in the upper body, an inexplicable bout of wakefulness in the night, some twitching or itching or aching joints, or whatever. It may be that in retrospect you later realized that other changes were taking place on other levels and you had not connected them. Perhaps a significant dream occurred. Often, when these nonphysical signs present themselves, we search around in our outer lives to find explanations. This must have happened because of such and such, we say. Outer changes may well be happening, for this is often a time of life that brings such outer changes. So we hitch the inner changes to those life events. It may well be that those outer events have had a triggering effect on the inner process. Who knows? If you have not already done this, take a moment to think about the possible, less obvious, inner events which may have occurred and consider that these, too, may have been part of the overall process of menopause, rather than chance happenings.

My menopause began with the dream of the woman on the gun carriage, but I was only dimly aware of that until the physical signs confirmed it. Maybe it is really only in retrospect that I knew the dream was the beginning. It is hard to know now.

For many of the women to whom I have spoken, the physical signs were the first ones they noticed. Such signs are often erratic periods, which may be lighter or heavier, irregular, stopping and starting, or in some other way changing the characteristic pattern they have held for all those menstruating years.

I remember that when my periods first began to dwindle and skip beats I felt a sense of panic at the realization that something so familiar would soon be ended forever. Not that I wanted to keep menstruating, for my days of procreation were well and truly over and I, like most other women, was glad to contemplate the end of all the inconvenience associated with bleeding. Nevertheless, I felt a sudden strangeness at the thought that it was really ending—a certain apprehensiveness about the change and all that it signified.

One day I suddenly realized I might never see my menstrual blood again. I began to cry. It was as though the full reality of it had hit me. Like leaving school, or arriving in a foreign country for the first time, there was that sinking feeling, knowing that the old, secure, familiar world was transforming into something else.

I wept, too, because I knew that for me to be able to come to terms with change, it would be really important to face up to it and feel it fully, and one of my ways to do that would be to create ritual, to act out the change in some way, on a symbolic level.

I found myself wishing that I had been able somehow to mark with a ritual that moment of my menstrual dying. I needed to see my blood again in order to say good-bye, and I realized that now, maybe, I never would. I needed to hold a funeral, but there was no body to bury. I was full of sadness and regret.

However, there was another period. The textbooks say that we have to be free of periods for at least a full year before we can say with assurance that we have "menopaused." So I bled again, of course. There was no way of knowing whether this was to be the last time, but I knew by then what I wanted to do. I took a smooth, white seashell and smeared the inside with my blood. Into the curved bowl of the upturned shell, now the color of womb-ochre, I placed three tiny, round pebbles. One was pure white, to symbolize the virgin, one rock red for the earth mother, and one pure black for the crone. I put them on my dresser to remind me. Now I was satisfied. The realization of what was happening in my body, the mourning, and the ritual, these three things completed a process, and I was ready to move on. From then on, the occasional appearances of blood seemed without significance, mere physical happenings requiring the necessary hygienic measures. They seemed far less central now, to my experience. The image of myself as a menstruating woman was leaving me, and leaving me ready for the next phase of my life.

In such a way we shuttle between the ordinary and the sacred, the practical and the symbolic aspects of living. Today my neighbor remarked upon the sky. It was one of those dramatic days, a bright blue heaven rich with extravagant, swirling cumulus clouds. My first thought was about the chance that it might rain on the washing that I had hung out to dry in the sun, and I felt ashamed of my reaction. Then I reflected that we had each seen one aspect of the sky, my neighbor and I, and simply shared them. There is no special merit in seeing one or the other. The merit is in being able to be open to both. The sacred and the profane. They are always hand in hand. Every human experience holds them both.

The trouble with the "medical model," the physician's way of conceptualizing menopause, is that it allows only for one aspect. Not that it concentrates totally on the physical, of course. Any doctor will admit that there are mental and emotional components of the menopausal change of life, but these are seen as extensions of the process in the same dimension, mental "symptoms" to be considered alongside the physical ones, perhaps even medicated. Inasmuch as medicine remains unaware of the spiritual aspects of the process, it renders it two-dimensional.

I believe that each of us has the right to experience our whole life in all three dimensions, which means acknowledging the spiritual aspect in everything. It is that spiritual dimension which has the power to bring each and every experience truly alive.

So many women with whom I have talked had no inkling of this other way of envisioning menopause. With childbirth, yes, or marriage, or death, the sacred dimension was clearly seen, but this other rite of passage, this special time, had no significance for many except in a practical sense.

The point about the sacred aspect is not simply that it adds beauty to everything we do, although in fact it often does. It is not simply frosting on an otherwise plain cake. The deeper function of the sacred is that it enables us to embrace our lives fully rather than hesitantly, eagerly rather than grudgingly. By creating for us a context in which every event of our lives has a meaning of some kind, it gives us the ability to take hold of those events and live them to the fullest of which we are capable.

As tourists, we flock hungrily to see and feel the cultures whose spiritual qualities are up-front and palpable. The Balinese culture, for example, where every moment of the waking day is imbued with meaning and ritual significance. Yet in our own culture, we starve for meaning. Like the textbook frog, who starves to death amid a pile of dead flies because he does not recognize his food unless it is on the wing, we starve amid plenty. We do not recognize that in every event, every moment, there is a sacred dimension to our being. Especially at those points in our lives where changes noticeably happen, we have a deep need to know that dimension, not only for its enriching, aesthetic qualities, but also as a way of understanding who we are, of interpreting the story of our lives and the events which are happening to and around us, a way of knowing what these times mean and how to live them.

Our society is not very good at creating rites of passage over and above the few very obvious ones. Subcultures within the main culture each have their own, of course. The Jewish culture is particularly rich with them. But for millions of people, there are few opportunities to engage in rituals with a true rite-of-passage quality, despite the many points in our lives when such rituals could ease us into change and celebrate the change process.

Life has so many transitions, and yet for so many of those transitional experiences "we have no rituals, no way of helping people make sense out of the apparent contradictions and senselessness of the new situation. There is no symbolic rite for giving up the family home, getting divorced, completing menopause, relinquishing one's driver's license."[1]

Of course, as we noted earlier, our ancestors often did not live long enough to see their own fertility end, so it is not surprising that anthropologists have failed to find menopause rituals from the past. But we need them now. This important period of change in a woman's life "is a change that needs symbolic interpretation. The need of the modern woman to find a symbolic framework for this fundamental stage of life is acute."[2]

As I mentioned in Chapter 2, the concept of the rite of passage was first put forward by the anthropologist van Gennep in his studies of life transitions in various tribal societies. He described rituals and ceremonies, often strictly observed, which marked the transition of an individual from one life stage to the next.[3]

The rite of passage is a symbolic bridging mechanism which enables a person's psyche to accept the transition from stage to stage. It has certain classic features. One generally finds that there is an element of withdrawal from the world, a withdrawal into that other, sacred dimension. This is the function of our cocoon. It is a vitally necessary part of our process if we are to experience our menopause as fully as we are able.

Another common element is that of ordeal. There is some kind of pain, some kind of burning or cutting which leaves its mark, impresses its point. We have only to think of the circumcision which is part of the rite of puberty for boys in many cultures to see a clear example of this. (I cannot bring myself to think of female circumcision in this light, although I know that in some sense it is, for the people who practice it. I am afraid I am able to see it only as a particularly horrifying form of oppression rather than a genuine rite of passage. I cannot believe that genuine rites of passage inflict lifelong, disabling mutilation which robs the participant of life's basic, normal functions.)

Menopause has its pain, its grieving, its mourning for what has gone, its confusion about what is now and what is to come. For many women, menopause is, at some level, an ordeal.

Then there is the return. This is when we emerge from the cocoon metamorphosed in such a way that we now know ourselves differently from the inside even if we appear the same to others on the outside. It is likely that we shall now have a new reference group, a new body of people with whom we have begun to identify.

As well as these elements—the withdrawal, the ordeal, and the return—rites of passage have another important aspect, which is that they are public events rather than private ones. Their power lies in the fact that they are an inescapable part of tribal culture, embedded in the experience of each person and in the history and tradition of the group. When we do encounter one of the rare rites in our own culture, such as the wedding, for example, we may become suddenly aware of the powerful force behind the tradition. One may have a feeling of being swept up into a process that is so much bigger than the individual and to a great extent beyond the power of the individual to influence.

This poses a problem. Menopause is virtually invisible in our society, just as menstruation itself has always been invisible. How, then, can we create a rite of passage which is public, one in which the group as a whole stands by to bear witness, to confirm the experience of the one who is passing through the transition?

Here and there some people, particularly women, are creating group rituals of their own. Knowing the power of the group experience, they are providing that opportunity for their members to underscore and honor the individual's important times of transition. This is a small beginning. Often, such groups are to be found in a subculture of women-identified women—those who have turned their back on the patriarchal culture as fully as they can. Already marginalized by the mainstream of their society, they feel the necessity to create their own forms. There is joy for women in such forms, since they are created specifically by and for women themselves.

Once again, however, these are a drop in the bucket when compared to the popular culture in its broadest sense, the modern, Western, materialist culture in which so many of us live and try to breathe.

Menopausal women are but one group which stands in need of a public rite of passage to mark, honor, and assist an inner change. Men, too, in many aspects of their lives, are lacking forms. Steven Foster, who has been working to create new puberty rites for young men in the modern spiritual vacuum, bemoans the fact that "a modern passage rite does not contain the full social force of a traditional one. At the present time our culture does not validate or focus on such rites." In order for this to happen, huge changes would have to take place.

> For a modern passage ceremony to gain the full power of an ancient one, the very drift of our culture towards secular materialism would have to be diverted. But given the reality of our culture, we can only start with what we have and work to create the best model possible under the circumstances.[4]

It seems to me that in order to prepare the way for a world in which such ceremonies are commonplace and in which the sacred dimension of ordinary life is known and touched by all, we must first learn to recontact the sacred in ourselves and bring it back into all that we do. First we must go within and listen to ourselves, to the messages arising from our bodies and from the deeper layers of our consciousness. Then we must learn to honor them, to grace them with ritual perhaps, if that feels appropriate.

There may be opportunities to create group rituals, group acknowledgments of our inner processes of change. Gradually, if we persist, new forms may arise. There probably is no other way to proceed except to start with ourselves and go from there.

As Robert Johnson points out in his teaching on ways to work with dreams, the acting out of our personal symbolism in the outer world in some way seems to validate it and make it real and solid. The lesson it teaches is then more thoroughly learned and integrated. He explains:

> Although we can understand the meaning of symbols with our minds, our understanding is made immeasurably deeper and more concrete when we *feel* the symbols with our bodies and our feelings. When we only think about symbols, or talk about them, we are able to detach ourselves too readily from the feeling quality that surrounds them. But if we *do* something

to express the symbol—something that involves our bodies and
our emotions—the symbol becomes a living reality for us. It
etches itself indelibly on our consciousness.[5]

I can speak only from my own private and group experience.
The insights and breakthroughs in understanding which came
from my inward probings were inevitably and invariably
made more useful and more meaningful by crystallizing them
in some outer action, however symbolic. My blood-smeared
seashell set with stones was for me a powerful tool to use in
coming to terms with the changes in my physiology. It aided
me in saying good-bye to the old and in starting to accept the
new.

Not everyone will do these things in the same way. It is
important that each of us do only that which seems to fit the
moment, the occasion, the person we feel ourselves to be. It
matters little what form our work takes. What we do inside
the cocoon is our own business entirely. Please do not take
my personal recipes as prescriptions for your own process,
unless of course they seem to fit. The really important thing
is to find what works and feels right for *you*.

In the same way, the postmenopausal woman you become
is in every way an individual. Her own person. Your way of
manifesting the crone may be completely different from mine,
and so it should be. That very freedom, the freedom to define
ourselves however we like, is central to the crone phase of our
lives more than at any other time.

So I hope that in some things you will question me, raise
your eyebrows, disagree. Your story, your formulation of menopause and what it means is as important and as valid as
mine. I just happen to have gone public in writing mine down
before it became a popular thing to do.

Your heroes and heroines may well be different from mine,
your experiences worlds away, your models polar opposites
of the ones that have been my inspiration. What I am urging
you to do is to consider who you are and what has shaped
you and to give a form and meaning to your menopause that
are all your own.

Perhaps if you have some time for reflection you could bring into your awareness some of the female images which have inspired you, particularly of late. To whose life story has your interest been drawn in fascination or in admiration?

Maybe there are women in history in whom you can see manifested the power and wisdom of the crone. They may be women of our own times, like Margaret Mead, whose own life seemed to embody the "menopausal zest" of which she spoke, or heroines of an earlier age, like Susan B. Anthony, whose zeal, unabated in her old age, won freedoms for all her sisters more than a decade after her own life had ended. They may be women of the distant past, or mythical women. The Goddesses of Olympus, perhaps, with their fantastic lives, endless situations that model our own, and ways of dealing with them that script us even now.

Recall what you know and feel of all the traditions, all the sources of wisdom that have affected you, whether by birth or simply by your own attraction to them. We all have an instinct which draws us unfailingly toward the myths and symbols, the models and rituals we need in order to give our lives the dimension of deep meaning. Furthermore, we have a hungry need for them. They are like the clues in a treasure hunt, the mysterious messages we must discover and read in order to find our way to where the treasure is. In the case of our real life journeys, the treasure is found by journeying inward, into our inner worlds. Myths and symbols are the clues that lead us beyond our everyday world by taking us, paradoxically, more and more deeply into it, into our own life experience. In the words of Joseph Campbell,

> People say that what we're all seeking is a meaning for life. I don't think that's what we're really seeking. I think that what we're seeking is an experience of being alive, so that our life experiences on the purely physical plane will have resonances within our own innermost being and reality, so that we actually feel the rapture of being alive. That's what it's all finally about, and that's what these clues help us to find within ourselves.[6]

What are your favorite stories? Who are your favorite Gods and Goddesses, saints and heroes? Whose biography excites you, inspires you? Who would you like to be like?

You may want to make up a story, a myth, or a fairy tale. Perhaps you want to draw or paint images of the Goddess, or compose a tune or song, a hymn or poem.

Have you made an altar? If not, would it feel good to make one? What are the objects that are special to you? Arrange them lovingly upon your altar.

Luisah Teish points out that although the idea of making an altar may seem strange to us, many of us do it unconsciously, not even realizing that is what we are doing:

> I am amazed at how much of what we call interior decorating is really just subconscious altar-building. I've been in homes of people who swear they are 'not the least bit spiritual,' yet I find Grandma's picture standing next to a lovely bouquet, on a hand-crocheted doily and a lamp nearby.[7]

Our choice of animal companions and images may be another unconscious manifestation of our inner magic. I work near a wisdom-proud professor, for example, whose office is decorated all over with owls, and a warm and free-spirited social worker of independent disposition who is one floor up from us in a room adorned with cats.

What are your companion creatures, your familiars, your power animals? What qualities do you see in the other creatures of the earth that draw you into a feeling of affinity? It may be the freedom and power of the eagle, the cleverness of the coyote, the strength of the bear.

What are the special symbols in your dreams? I dreamed once of a silver crocodile. Some time later, I wrote a story about him. It was a story that seemed to come out of some deep place inside me, a story that wrote itself. When I read the story later, it was full of meaning for me, telling me things about myself that I had never realized before. When the images in your dreams have that special, numinous quality that seems to follow you into your waking day, that haunting specialness that feels different and important, then turn toward them and listen to what they have to say. Capture them on paper or in clay, perhaps, or dance them. Play with them. Let them unfold their meanings to you. This is your private magic.

If you care to share it, it can be shared. I am finding even deeper meaning in my own magic as I go through the exercise of sharing it with you, here, now.

The caricature of the crone which has come down to us is the witch, hunched over her cauldron, weaving wicked spells with which to do her mischief in the world. That image, so familiar to all of us from our childhood books, is all that is left of the wise crone in our popular culture. Yet once we understand the past, we can reconstruct the powerful images that had become lost to us, just as the archeologists reconstitute a whole, lost culture from a pile of dusty shards. The witch's cave is her cocoon. This is where she retreats to do her all-important inner work, and it is from here that she will fly to take her wisdom out where it is needed, in large ways or in small. Her cat is by her side, lone representative of the world of creatures and co-opted powers, feelings, and natural processes. Her book, her cauldron, all the ritual things she uses are her power objects. It is they who deepen her experience, strengthen her wisdom, equip her for her work. Mischief she can create, but probably she will not want to unless she is split off, discounted, uninvited to the wedding. Then she will become bitter; her anger will grow and her power will seem threatening. If she is accepted, welcomed, reunited with the other aspects of the archetypal female, her power is for healing and her wisdom is for sharing.

Begin to know her. Take a journey to her cave. Befriend her and become her, for you are she and she is you. In whatever ways are right for you, do your share of reclaiming the crone, for all our sakes. You may want to paint her, or to model her in clay. You may prefer to find pictures and images that express her for you. Perhaps you want to write about her or to read as much as you can about her history—or, as they say, her herstory—and how her power was lost to our world for so many centuries. Now it is being reclaimed, and you and I are part of that reclamation. Even if we do nothing more in our lives except let ourselves enter fully into that power, we shall have done something important for all men and women everywhere, and for the planet itself. An ancient balance is gradually being restruck.

Find things which symbolize her and put them on your altar. See her face in the mirror and talk with it. You may need to face a lot of fear and pain in order to get to her. What we are speaking of here is not a movie script, a sentimental tale to be enjoyed and forgotten. It is real life, and it can hurt.

Coming to terms with Kali is not simply getting used to the sight of one's advancing wrinkles. Neither does she represent "some abstract idea of an everlasting death and rebirth cycle which we can watch from a safe vantage-point and affirm. We are talking about our own nitty-gritty finitude."[8] These bodies and minds in which we live and move will one day die. With them will go our dreams. We shall take leave of our relationships for the last time, and those who love us and whom we love will mourn as they burn or bury in the earth this flesh that now is warm and alive. Oh yes, Kali's breath on our necks is real, and it is cold. We must fully feel the pain of our finitude, our mortality, before we can truly aspire to our title of crone.

Once we have faced this pain, however, once we have let ourselves be drawn all the way to the bottom of the vortex, like Innana in the underworld,[9] then there is a change, a transformation. The spiraling in will begin to give way to a spiraling out again, out into the world.

In facing the ultimate fear, the fear of annihilation, we enable ourselves to move beyond it. When one "gives in to finitude," says Rita Gross, "a softer lighter touch can be expected." Here, again, is the lightness of which we spoke in the previous chapter.

> There is an immense relief and release and consequent bubbling over of spontaneous energy. Tremendous strength and a new, less problematic relation to suffering result. One might say there is a kind of imperturbable calm, whatever the situation. The indestructibility permits a gentle and powerfully effective mode of relationship with the world.[10]

Just as it is important to pay homage to the sacred dimension in ordinary, everyday moments and happenings, so it is also important, I believe, to ground our "spiritual" experiences in normality and ordinariness.

In my work, I have met many people, both men and women, whose pursuit of the spiritual seems to me to have led them away from real life rather than toward it. I agree, of course, that there is sometimes a place for asceticism as a vehicle for awakening one's awareness. The practice of various kinds of abstinence, such as fasting, for example, serves an important cleansing function at certain times, most surely leads to heightened levels of sensitivity, and may facilitate altered states of consciousness, if these are being sought. However, my personal belief is that a fully human life, lived out on all levels, physical, mental, emotional, spiritual, is the greatest, albeit most difficult, thing we can achieve, and also the greatest praise we can offer to whatever God we have.

I agree with Starhawk when she says,

> It is easier to be celibate than to be fully alive sexually. It is easier to withdraw from the world than to live in it; easier to be a hermit than to raise a child; easier to repress emotions than to feel them and express them; easier to meditate in solitude than to communicate in a group; easier to submit to another's authority than place trust in oneself. It is not easy to be a Witch.[11]

Neither is it easy to live menopause in the way I am suggesting we live it. For one thing, there are others to consider.

It is not always easy to explain the cocoon to those around us. Remember Marie, in Chapter 6, whose reassessment of her priorities "rocked the boat at home"? There are many like Marie whose new demand for time and space of their own creates consternation in the others with whom they share their daily lives. Families and other households tend to operate like mobiles, delicately balanced. Change one part of the system and the whole system is affected in some way. The balance changes. The folk we live with adapt to our routines and we to theirs, however subtle those routines might be, so when someone's routine changes, even very slightly, there is an effect on the others.

Of course, we are not obliged to give explanations. If we have chosen to rearrange our time a little, or to change our routine way of doing things, it is sufficient that we simply announce the change to anyone who may be affected in some way by it. It seems only fair to tell those affected that there is to be a change, but we owe no one an explanation of our private, inner processes.

We may choose to attempt it, nonetheless. In intimate relationships, the intimacy is deepened whenever we are enabled, by the empathic caring of our partners, to reveal and share our deepest selves. It is not necessary that our partners should be able to understand, totally. the experience which we are sharing. It is sufficient that they listen, that they care, and that they accept.

Several lesbian women have told me that they believe menopause is easier for them than for heterosexual women, since it is easier for a woman to understand another woman's experience. They can share fully with their partners, knowing that what they say will resonate somewhere inside the partner's psyche also.

To a certain extent, this holds true for all our relationships with other women, whether sexual or not. Of all the women whose menopause experiences I have studied, a vast majority have told me that they turn, above all, to other women when they want to talk or ask about these matters. They turn to friends, mothers, sisters, colleagues, daughters, seeking that resonance, that shared understanding of what it means to inhabit a woman's body and live a woman's life.

Among those who have male partners, there are those who try to share it and those who do not. I was one who did, and my attempts have been abundantly rewarded. For one thing, I have discovered that in my efforts to explain my inner experiences of menopause to someone who has no prior knowledge of such things, I have made them clearer to myself.

I also have found that in our stumbling attempts to understand the mysteries of yin and yang, of male and female ways of being and how to harmonize them, my sharing of my deepest female processes has called forth in my male partner a parallel sharing of his deep male ones. To a degree which has surprised me, he has been able to understand and empathize, and also to confront me ruthlessly when it was needed. He has been more fully able to relate to all the aspects of me, the virgin, the mother, and the crone, simply because I have been more aware of them myself and have shown them to him.

It is only because of the trust in this particular relationship that such a sharing has been possible. It is not so with all relationships. It would not have been possible for me in my first marriage, for example. Not because my previous partner would not have understood—in face he has a vast capacity for understanding such issues—but because in those days I was not yet ready to trust enough. I was not yet ready to let myself be unconditionally vulnerable. At this time, with this partner, I am.

So to whom do you talk about menopause? Maybe you have spoken with your women friends, or your relatives. Maybe you have shared it with your partner, if you have one. Perhaps you prefer to talk to no one. You must do whatever feels right for you. Let no one tell you how it should be. Let no one else define it but you. And let even your own definitions be flexible, variable, changeable. One day it may be serious, heavy, deeply introspective. The next day it may be light, free, funny. Let it be whatever it is, in each moment. If we can learn to let our definitions be fluid and unfixed, to change shape, like clouds change even as we watch them, we may eventually learn to live without definitions altogether one day. Who knows? This is the lightness of the crone, the witch, the shape-shifter. Travelling through life without excess baggage.

That reminds me of another fantasy I have. This is the fantasy that as I age I shall gradually, slowly, divest myself of more and more material possessions, thus paralleling the inner process of lightening with an outer one. I have seen older women doing this, and it has always seemed extraordinarily appropriate. However, as yet I am unable to do it myself. There always seems to be a reason for keeping everything. The minute I go to throw something out, I think of a use for it!

What are your fantasies of growing older? What are the tasks you see ahead of you? Who are the women you have watched and from whom you have learned? What sort of an old woman are you going to be? Regardless of our attempts to divine it, the future remains, by definition, an unplanned adventure, a mapless trail, leading toward an unknown destination. We can have hopes, plans, dreams, ideals, even expectations. But we must carry them lightly, being prepared to let them go at any and every moment, and to surrender into change and unknowing. This is the way of true aliveness.

* * *

Menopause is a universal female experience. It is a stage in the life of each woman which marks the end of the second segment of her life journey and the beginning of her entrance to the third. As such, it has the potential to be an important rite of passage, an outer event which may be consciously used to assist an inner process. This is the spirit in which I have talked about menopause throughout these pages.

For many people, this will be a new way of thinking about the matter. Our culture, for the most part, sees menopause as a clinical event—a simple, biological happening which, for certain people, has emotional "side effects."

Medicine has found an opportunity to involve itself, and drug companies make profits from the sale of hormones. The subject of biological menopause is scientifically complicated, and it is hard to steer a course through those waters.

I have tried to go a different way. From the starting point of my own experience, I have explored the deeper significance of menopause, the emotional, psychological, and spiritual meanings it may hold, and its transformative potential, both for the individual and for her society—and ultimately the whole planet. I have examined the way we feel in our female bodies, the changes that may come to our thinking and our feeling, the issues we have to face, and the fullness of development which I believe may be the result of living this key period of our lives with heightened awareness on all levels of our being.

Many women of my own generation have looked askance at my ideas, dismissing them as "a lot of fuss about nothing." For them, the ability to "sail through" this time of their lives, making as little of it as possible, has been seen as a sort of triumph. I would not want to take that from them. There

seems to be, however, a noticeable change in the attitudes of
the generation which is following. I am speaking of the generation of my younger sisters, and my younger friends, women
ten or fifteen years younger than me, whose menopause is just
coming on to the horizon. In many of these younger women,
there is a new spiritual hunger, a new desire to find personal
meaning and to re-vision the world's wisdom traditions in
ways that have modern relevance. It is from the ranks of this
age group, for example, that the women's spirituality movement finds some of its most articulate voices and the male
power structures in traditional religions are being challenged.
It is through them, I believe, and from the younger ones who
see and hear them, that crone wisdom is finding its way back
into a world which has long suppressed it.

It is in this group that I place the most hope for change.
The earth needs the power and energy of these women in order
to change the direction which has brought its outer layers—
the ecosystems of which we form a part—close to destruction.
If changes of direction in human affairs do not soon take effect,
our earth will have no choice but to let these layers go. It will
undress down to its bare rock and keep whirling into the
future without us.

As wise crones, we hold vast amounts of wisdom, and the
power to use that wisdom where it is needed. As crones, we
have become fully developed women—women who have come
to the full fruiting of their potential. From this fullness, we
can take our rightful place as equal partners in the spiritual
leadership of the world. We can teach men and learn from
them, and together make the repairs which are so desperately
needed. This fruiting is a spiritual harvest which I believe is
already beginning. I see it in the words and pictures and
experiences of women who are finally releasing the old bonds
and becoming fully free of old conditioning. These are the
women who, for the first time, are experiencing the complete-
ness of womanhood, in all its aspects. These are the women
who are living their menopause instead of "getting through"
it. They will live their old age, too, instead of getting through
that, and the world will know they are there. Not that they
will necessarily have to do anything in particular. They will

simply be who they are. After their spiraling inward and their
period of time in the cocoon, they will once again spiral outward, coming to live in the world in a new way, light and
wise. The way in which they live may not look dramatically
different. It is the inner change which counts. If the inner
ripening has taken place, then the power and wisdom of the
crone is within them and it may manifest in a million different
ways, some of them very, very subtle.

When older women are able to live out fully, in their lives,
the archetypal power of the crone, then younger women will
have greater and greater access to that crone aspect of themselves which is already there in some measure.

I am limited by who I am and have been. What I have tried
to do, however, is tell my story and open up my ideas so that
they create an opportunity for you to tell your own story.
There must be so many other ways of understanding these
things, so many other ways of living menopause and being a
woman, so many other ways of finding meaning.

You will have your own ways, your own metaphors. I have
given you some of mine. Many of them are organic ones, concerned with growth. As I said at the beginning, growth is a
powerful metaphor for all of us in this culture. It has also
been a common motif for many of the women who, at my
request, have drawn pictures of their menopause.

After the rosebud comes the rose. And after the rose petals
wither and fall there is a period of waiting. Then one day, if
we are patient, we notice a full, red rosehip on the end of the
stem. Rosehips are beautiful in their own way. They are tough
and long-lasting and are full of vitamin C, but many people
never wait to see them. They simply prune the dead roses to
make the garden look neater. The flower dies and falls and we
say, "What a shame," and look for another. I used to wonder
what lay beyond prime time, and now I think I know. An
undervalued fruit. My book has been about this crone fruit
and how we might ripen and harvest it.

There are some, like Susan, whose petals never open in any
way that I can understand, and yet at some level their lives
have meaning, I have no doubt. These are the things which
puzzle us when we try to probe the mysteries of living. Beyond

all our knowing, there is always the unknown. To accept that is to make the ultimate surrender. It is the surrender which brings us, finally, into wisdom.

The first step in learning surrender is to spiral inward, in toward the unknown center of the self. For in there, if we brave the darkness, is the beginning of the path which can lead us out again into the light.

Thank you, Susan, for the metaphor.

EPILOGUE: FREE AS A
BUTTERFLY

Is there one definitive moment when the cocoon breaks open and we emerge into the light? One epiphanal experience that leaves us forever transformed?

I believe that the answer to this question is both yes and no. "Yes," because we do experience deeply symbolic moments in our lives which leave us feeling irrevocably changed: like the first bleeding, the loss of virginity, the day the last child leaves home, retirement, death of a parent, and so on. There are many such thresholds in the course of one woman's lifetime. Once we step over one of these, there is no going back. We are changed, whether we like it or not, and often in the space of a few minutes or hours. There may certainly be moments, especially in the menopausal years, when we have the distinct sense of emerging from a cocoon into the light, with wet wings, and seeing the world in a new way. I have felt like this from time to time, and maybe you have, too.

"No," because usually we have to learn to *live* the change. We have to practice being who we newly are. It does not come easily or automatically, as a rule.

If you tune in to your inner processes, as this book has suggested, this menopausal stage of life may contain a number of deeply symbolic and transformative moments which you will recognize. Inner work, particularly creative imagination, dreamwork, meditation, and the exercises we have discussed here, such as dancing, singing, and illustrating one's inner issues, tends to produce such highly meaningful moments for many people. These arise in the course of the work itself and sometimes spontaneously at other times, too, as a result of the heightened awareness which the work encourages.

These experiences cannot stand alone, however. They need to be embodied, brought to life, grounded in everyday functioning. They have to be integrated into our total being, made a part of our ordinary lives. Only then can we truly say that we are out of the cocoon.

Menopause, when it occurs naturally, is often a very gradual process, spread over a long time, usually several years. The actual cessation of the menstrual periods is an event which can only be recognized retrospectively. Unless we are preparing for a hysterectomy, there is no way we can knowingly remove the last tampon and say, "That's it!" It is more likely that, after being accustomed to erratic or infrequent periods, we shall one day look around and realize that there has been no bleeding for a whole year and we are officially "menopaused," biologically at least, though hot flashes may continue for a long time.

Likewise, there may be a day when we look around and suddenly notice that the feelings and sensations which used to characterize the menopausal life stage have gently given way to a lighter, calmer, and more mellow way of being and that our long, slow emergence from the cocoon is complete. We have become, as Mary Daly would say, a "Free/wild Crone."[1]

What is the nature of this new woman? For each of us, the answer will be different, since each of us is unique. To the extent that one can generalize, here are some of the qualities which I believe the new woman may have.

Freed from so many of her previous roles and limiting definitions, this woman may at times seem bold. Bold, that is, in a special and often enviable way. She may develop the habit of cutting through pretense and pomposity and going straight to the heart of things. She does not do this from any desire to shock, for her boldness is not a device of the attention-seeking ego. It has more in common with the simple honesty of a child; an honesty freed from the constraints of worrying about what other people will think.

After two-thirds of a lifetime spent in rehearsing for the future and holding endless postmortems on the dead body of the ever-imperfect past, she may finally have learned the art of staying in the present. She may understand, at last, how wonderful it feels to live in the moment, in the eternal, endless NOW.

Naturally, even though she knows how wonderful it is, she may not always remember to do it. However, she may be less hard on herself for forgetting and for lapsing into the old habits. In fact, she may be less hard on herself all round, and on others, too. Maybe she will have begun to accept herself for who and what she is—and is not. In this accepting of herself in the round, without splitting and judgment, she may also have learned to accept others in the same way.

Maybe she will laugh a lot because who she is—or thought she was—does not matter a whole lot and she has finally realized that. Even though she may have known it in her head for a long time, and probably read it in 100 books and heard it from the lips of at least a dozen teachers, she now knows it all the way down. It is part of her being now.

I expect this will be just one of the many things she has known in her head for a long time and is now feeling inside her. There is a wisdom in her now which she can neither locate nor explain. Sometimes she will open her mouth and words will come out, and she will listen in faint surprise, wondering from whence they come. She does not always know the value of the gift she gives; thus other people's reactions may surprise her sometimes. She wonders why they value her so highly, for, like LeGuin's "space crone," she feels so "ordinary."[2]

She may think she has forgotten a lot of her knowledge, and indeed she probably has, but it matters less and less. It is her wisdom the world needs now, rather than her knowledge. Often the younger people have a monopoly on knowledge anyhow. She is learning to accept that, knowing that she still has her library card, for use when needed. Let other people update the knowledge files! She will consult one if she needs it, for she still remembers how to use the catalogue.

Knowledge is always there but wisdom has to be created. It is created from the raw material of a lifetime of experience and transmuted, like the menstrual blood which no longer flows, into the special, precious wisdom of the crone. That rich, female experience which has filled her inner spaces has changed into the wisdom which she will give back to the world around her. Her blood has become wisdom now and she will give it more and more, becoming lighter and finer even as she does so. This is the harvest of her life. This is her alchemist's gold, created from the ordinariness of living and fired in the crucible of menopause.

Her giving is not in the old, selfless way of the mother, putting others' needs first the way women seem naturally to do,[3] for she gives generously to herself, too, whatever is needed. She does not deny herself or put herself last. She cannot afford to. She must husband her energy carefully, cherishing the body which still contains her. But she gives easily, since what she wants for herself is not a lot, now. It is only simple needs which have to be filled, rather than desires. She has finally learned to tell the difference.

There is lightness in her laughter, in the simplicity of her joys; lightness in the way she lives her life, taking little, giving where needed. There is a new lightness in her step, and her footprints in the earth are less deep now. There is also a glowing passion for living, a sparkle in the eye, and an energy that is clear and focused. The wisdom she gives to the world is distilled from her own living and from the knowledge she has processed and probably forgotten as well as that which she happens to remember. She may say, with Florida Scott-Maxwell, "My answers must be my own, years of reading now lost in the abyss I call my mind. What matters is what I have now, what in fact I live and feel."[4]

That living and that feeling may tire her more easily than in earlier days. But that does not stop her from using the energy she has. As Scott-Maxwell, writing in her eighties, said as she chronicled her own surges of crone energy, "all this is very tiring, but love at any age takes everything you've got."[5]

By entering into the fire of her own menopause, she has become better acquainted with burning. Pain and death no longer frighten her. If her body has ills, she bears them with fortitude and asks them humbly for the lessons they have to offer. Through her own learning, she can teach. Not necessarily in any formal kind of way, however. She teaches by simply being who she is.

* * *

A new powerfulness is stirring. There is a new sense of confidence in the air, and intimations of the hidden richness in postmenopausal life. I have found this sense of power and confidence and this deep and unexpected richness in the words and pictures of so many women.

Marie, the rocker of the family boat, whom we met in Chapter 6, gives us her own picture of the emerging crone: "A woman who has accepted menopause and moved on to me is a richer person. She displays a wisdom, a weathering endurance, inner beauty, an ageless quality." This woman has, for Marie, a "well of wisdom and strength."

We met Joan and Anne in Chapter 5. Joan was coming to terms with the issues of sexuality and aging; Anne was lamenting the loss of her childbearing potential, even though her family was long since complete. In both of them, a sense of the new power is beginning to show.

For Joan, it comes through in her readiness to take up her new vocation. She is moving beyond her nursing role to embrace other forms of working with people, including massage and spiritual counseling: "I feel more ready to assume my real work and destiny with a strong sense of purpose. I also feel people are more likely to accept spiritual wisdom from an older woman."

Anne has used her struggle about the end of fertility to distill her own brand of crone wisdom. Says Anne,

> This change in productivity is from the biological to the spiritual—a sense that comes from our years of childbearing and living. There is no degree, there is no school where wisdom can be bequeathed. Only the life process, and in this case the process of being fertile, of conceiving and bearing children and of becoming infertile but seeing your own children becoming

fertile.... I am a small part of the life force and this new phase
is also rich in a quiet and full way.... I can witness the mystery
of life but in no way can I control life.

Each of us is changing. Each of us is discovering, in her own
way, what lies beyond prime time. Each of us is finding her
own means to embody the qualities of the crone and to bring
them into the world. It is an ongoing journey of discovery for
us all.

* * *

There may be more I could say. But I cannot say it until I
discover it.

This part of my journey—the menopausal transition—began with my awareness of the inward-turning spiral. That
spiral, which was for me a symbol of all the changes I was
experiencing, seemed at first a frightening concept. My memory of the autistic child, Susan, who drew spirals all day, was
a memory of hopelessness and entrapment. It seemed the an-
tithesis of growth, and I believed so much in growth.

By entering into that vortex and surrendering to life as it
was being lived in me at that time, I came gradually to redefine all my ideas about what growth was, and is. I still
cannot explain why Susan's life had to be the way it was, nor
am I any closer to understanding how it might have seemed
to her. But at least I have been able to give up my crippling
need to make sense of it, for I have realized that my need to
make sense of everything has all my life been a thin disguise
for my need to control everything: a need to control which
grew from fear. This, I believe, is a fear we all share, the fear
of surrender into the process of life. By going into that inward
spiral, that vortex, I finally learned true surrender. I thought
I knew it before, but I knew it only with my intellect. I had
never experienced it in totality until the changes of menopause began to happen and I began to deal with them by
going into them instead of contracting from them. Menopause, for me, has truly been a spiritual journey.

Surrender, I have discovered, is not a on-off act. It is a
contract with life, renewed in each moment. It is a continual

process of free-fall. The new woman who is me is being re-
made, moment by moment. What I tell you about her now
may be out of date by the end of the day, or even by the end
of this page.

So this journey continues. It has no end. Join me.

NOTES

INTRODUCTION: THE INWARD SPIRAL

1. Ursula Leguin, "The Space Crone," *Co-Evolution Quarterly* 10 (July 21, 1976): p. 110.

1. WHAT IS MENOPAUSE?

1. Joel Wilbush, "What's in a Name? Some Linguistic Aspects of the Climacteric," *Maturitas* 3 (1981): pp. 1–9.

2. Carl Jung, *Collected Works* Vol. 8, paras. 784–787 (edited by Sir H. Read et al. Bollingen Series 20, Princeton, NJ: Princeton University Press, 1954).

3. Wulf Utian, *The Menopause in Modern Perspective: A Guide to Clinical Practice* (New York: Appleton-Century-Crofts, 1980), p. 18.

4. Yewoubdar Beyene, "Cultural Significance and Physiological Manifestations of Menopause: A Biocultural Analysis," *Culture, Medicine & Psychiatry* 10 (1986): pp. 47–71.

5. Ibid., p. 61.

6. Joel Wilbush, "Climacteric Expression & Social Context," *Maturitas* 4 (1982): p. 203 (n. 33).

7. Margaret Mead, *Male and Female: A Study of the Sexes in a Changing World* (New York: William Morrow, 1949), p. 229.

8. Joel Wilbush, 1982, p. 200.

9. Ibid., p. 199.

10. E. Trinkaus and D. Thompson, "Femoral Diaphyseal Histomorphometric Age Determinations for the Shanidar 3, 4, 5 & 6 Neandertals and Neandertal Longevity," *American Journal of Physical Anthropology* Vol. 72 (1987): pp. 123–129.

11. W. Gifford-Jones, MD, *On Being a Woman: The Modern Woman's Guide to Gynaecology* (New York: Macmillan, 1971), p. 22.

172 NOTES

12. Patricia Kaufert and Penny Gilbert, "Women, Menopause and Medicalization," *Culture, Medicine & Psychiatry* 10 (1986): pp. 7–21.
13. See, for example, Sadja Greenwood's *Menopause, Naturally: Preparing for the Second Half of Life* (San Francisco: Volcano Press, 1984).
14. Margaret Lock, "Models and Practice in Medicine: Menopause as Symptom or Life Transition?" *Culture, Medicine & Psychiatry* 6 (1982): pp. 261–280.
15. P. A. Van Keep et al., eds., assisted by P. Freebody, *The Controversial Climacteric*, Workshop moderators' reports presented at the 3rd International Congress on Menopause, held in Ostend, Belgium, under the auspices of the International Menopause Society in 1981 (Lancaster, England: MTP Press, 1981), p. 27.

2. WHO AM I? WHAT AM I MADE OF?

1. Paula Weideger, *Menstruation and Menopause* (New York: Delta, 1977).
2. Judy Chicago, *Through the Flower: My Struggle as a Woman Artist* (New York: Doubleday, 1975), p. 135.
3. Arnold van Gennep, *The Rites of Passage* (trans. Vizedom, M. B. and G. L. Caffee, Chicago: University of Chicago Press, 1960).
4. Joseph Campbell, *Myths to Live By* (New York: Bantam, 1975), p. 47.
5. Esther Harding, *Women's Mysteries Ancient and Modern* (New York: Harper & Row, 1971), p. 68.
6. Penelope Shuttle and Peter Redgrove, *The Wise Wound: Eve's Curse and Everywoman: Menstruation as a Powerful and Positive Resource in the Life of Women* (New York: Richard Marek, 1978).
7. Margaret Mead, *Male and Female*, p. 181.
8. Richard Moss, MD, *The Black Butterfly: An Invitation to Radical Aliveness* (Berkeley, CA: Celestial Arts, 1986), p. 275.

3. WHO AM I? WHAT DO I THINK?

1. Fritz Perls, *Gestalt Therapy Verbatim* (New York: Bantam, 1970), p. 53.
2. Thomas Berry, *The Dream of the Earth* (San Francisco: Sierra Club, 1988), p. 215.
3. A good text for understanding the differences in function between the cerebral hemispheres is Robert Ornstein's *The Psychology of Consciousness* (New York: Penguin, 1972).
4. For a succinct explanation of Jung's four functions, I recommend *The Portable Jung*, edited by Joseph Campbell (New York: Penguin, 1975).
5. *The Gospel According to Thomas: The Gnostic Sayings of Jesus* (trans. Guillaumont et al., New York: Harper & Row, 1984), Log. 22.
6. Aldous Huxley, *The Perennial Philosophy* (New York: Harper & Row, 1945).
7. Idries Shah, *Learning How to Learn: Psychology and Spirituality in the Sufi Way* (San Francisco: Harper & Row, 1981), p. 64.

4. WHO AM I? WHAT DO I FEEL?

1. See Chapter 4 of *The Portable Jung* for an explanation of the collective unconscious.
2. Robert Johnson, *Inner Work: Using Dreams and Active Imagination for Personal Growth* (New York: Harper & Row, 1986). In this useful book, Johnson describes ways of working with dreams that seek out our own personal meanings for the images our sleeping minds create, for extending our dream-work into our waking day, and for integrating this unconscious material into the everyday reality of our lives.

5. TIME OF TRANSITION: THE COMMON THEMES OF MENOPAUSE

1. William Bridges, *Transitions: Making Sense of Life's Changes* (Reading, MA: Addison-Wesley, 1980).
2. Ann Mankowitz, *Change of Life: A Psychological Study of Dreams and the Menopause* (Toronto, Canada: Inner City Books, 1984), p. 105.
3. Ibid., p. 106.
4. Elissa Melamed, *Mirror, Mirror: The Terror of Not Being Young* (New York: Linden Press, Simon and Schuster, 1983), p. 11.

6. WHO AM I REALLY?

1. Wulf Utian, *Your Middle Years: A Doctor's Guide for Today's Woman* (New York: Appleton-Century-Crofts, 1980), p. 85.
2. Lillian Rubin, *Women of a Certain Age: The Mid-Life Search for Self* (New York: Harper & Row, 1979).
3. Genia Pauli Hadden, *Body Metaphors: Releasing God-Feminine in Us All* (New York: Crossroads, 1988).
4. Erik Erikson, *Childhood and Society* (New York: W. W. Norton, 1950), p. 106.

7. WHO AM I BECOMING?

1. Merlin Stone, *When God Was a Woman* (New York: Harvest/HBJ, 1978), p. 1.
2. Naomi Goldenberg, *Changing of the Gods: Feminism and the End of Traditional Religions* (Boston: Beacon Press, 1979), p. 89.
3. Jean Shinoda Bolen, *Goddesses in Everywoman* (New York: Harper Colophon, 1985).
4. Barbara Walker, *The Crone: Woman of Age, Wisdom and Power* (New York: Harper & Row, 1985), p. 82.
5. Erich Neumann, *The Great Mother: An Analysis of the Archetype* (Trans. R. Mannheim, Bollingen, Series XLVII, Princeton, NJ: Princeton University Press, 1963), pp. 233/4.
6. Ibid., p. 229.
7. Genia Pauli Hadden, *Body Metaphors*, p. 160.

8. Nelle Morton, "The Goddess as Metaphoric Image," Plastow, J., and Christ, C., eds., *Weaving the Visions: New Patterns in Feminist Spirituality* (New York: Harper & Row, 1989), p. 113.

9. Pat Moore, "Gray Like Me: A Young Woman's Experiment with Aging," *New Age Journal* (March/April 1988).

10. Erik Erikson et al., *Vital Involvement in Old Age: The Experience of Old Age in Our Time* (New York: W. W. Norton, 1986), p. 294.

11. Simone de Beauvoir, *The Second Sex* (trans. H. M. Parshley, New York: Alfred Knopf, 1971), p. 583.

12. L. E. Troll et al., *Looking Ahead: A Woman's Guide to the Problems and Joys of Growing Older* (Englewood Cliffs, NJ: Prentice-Hall, 1977), p. 7.

13. Adrienne Rich, *Of Woman Born: Motherhood as Experience and Institution* (New York: Bantam, 1977), p. 86.

14. Linda Schierse Leonard, *The Wounded Woman: Healing the Father-Daughter Relationship* (Boulder, CO: Shambhala, 1983), p. 171.

15. Elissa Melamed, *Mirror, Mirror*, p. 17.

16. Stephanie Demetrakopoulos, "Life Stage Theory, Gerontological Research and the Mythology of the Older Woman: Independence, Autonomy and Strength," *Anima* 8/2, (1982): p. 93.

17. Simone de Beauvoir, *The Second Sex*, Chapter 20.

18. Ibid., p. 586.

19. Ibid., p. 590.

8. LIVING THE MENOPAUSE

1. C. Tavris, ed., *Everywoman's Emotional Wellbeing, Heart and Mind, Body and Soul* (New York: Doubleday, 1986), p. 247.

2. Penelope Washbourn, *Becoming Woman: The Quest for Wholeness in Female Experience* (New York: Harper & Row, 1977), p. 132.

3. Arnold Van Gennep, *The Rites of Passage*.

4. Steven Foster, "Passage into Manhood: A Modern Ritual for Young Men," *In Context* 16 (Spring 1987): pp. 50–54.

5. Robert Johnson, *Inner Work*, p. 103.

6. Joseph Campbell, *The Power of Myth* with Bill Moyers (New York: Doubleday, 1989), p. 5.

7. Luisah Teish, "Ancestor Reverence," *Weaving the Visions*, p. 90.

8. Rita Gross, "Suffering, Feminist Theory and Images of Goddess," *Anima* 13/1 (1986): p. 44.

9. The ancient Sumerian tale of Innana, one of the world's oldest recorded myths, was written in cuneiform on clay tablets in 1700 B.C. Beautifully retold by Sylvia Perera in her book *Descent to the Goddess: A Way of Initiation for Women* (Toronto, Canada: Inner City Books, 1981), it may be seen to symbolize woman's journey into the dark areas of the personal and collective unconscious.

10. Rita Gross, p. 42.

11. Starhawk, *The Spiral Dance: A Rebirth of the Ancient Religion of the Great Goddess* (San Francisco: Harper & Row, 1979), p. 197.

EPILOGUE: FREE AS A BUTTERFLY

1. Mary Daly, *Gyn-Ecology: The Metaethics of Radical Feminism* (Boston: Beacon Press, 1978), p. 249.

2. Ursula LeGuin, *The Space Crone*.

3. See, for example, Jean Baker Miller, *Towards a New Psychology of Women* (Boston: Beacon Press, 1976), for a full discussion of this alleged tendency.

4. Florida Scott-Maxwell, *The Measure of My Days* (New York: Alfred A. Knopf, 1968), p. 7.

5. Ibid., p. 13.

BIBLIOGRAPHY

Beauvoir, Simone de. *The Second Sex*, trans. H. M. Parshley. New York: Alfred Knopf, 1971.

Berry, Thomas. *The Dream of the Earth*. San Francisco: Sierra Club, 1988.

Beyene, Yewoubdar. "Cultural Significance and Physiological Manifestations of Menopause: A Biocultural Analysis." *Culture, Medicine & Psychiatry* 10, no. 1 (March 1986): pp. 47–71.

Bolen, Jean Shinoda. *Goddesses in Everywoman*. New York: Harper Colophon, 1985.

Bridges, William. *Transitions: Making Sense of Life's Changes*. Reading, MA: Addison-Wesley, 1980.

Campbell, Joseph. *Myths to Live By*. New York: Bantam, 1975.

———, with Bill Moyers. *The Power of Myth*. New York: Doubleday, 1988.

———, ed. *The Portable Jung*. New York: Penguin, 1975.

Castillejo, Irene C. de. *Knowing Woman*. New York: Harper Colophon, 1973.

Chicago, Judy. *Through the Flower: My Struggle as a Woman Artist*. New York: Doubleday, 1975.

Christ, Carol P. *Laughter of Aphrodite: Reflections on a Journey to the Goddess*. New York: Harper & Row, 1987.

———, and Plaskow, Judith, eds. *Womanspirit Rising: A Feminist Reader in Religion*. San Francisco: Harper & Row, 1979.

Colegrave, Sukie. *Uniting Heaven and Earth*. Los Angeles: Jeremy P. Tarcher, 1979.

Daly, Mary. *Gyn/Ecology: The Metaethics of Radical Feminism*. Boston: Beacon Press, 1978.

Demetrakopoulos, Stephanie A. "Life Stage Theory, Gerontological Research and the Mythology of the Older Woman: Independence, Autonomy and Strength." *Anima* 8, no. 2 (1982): 84–97.

———. *Listening to Our Bodies: The Rebirth of Feminine Wisdom*. Boston: Beacon Press, 1983.

Downing, Christine. *The Goddess: Mythological Images of the Feminine.* New York: Crossroad, 1981.
————. *Journey Through Menopause: A Personal Rite of Passage.* New York: Crossroad, 1987.
Erikson, Erik. *Childhood and Society.* New York: W. W. Norton, 1950.
————, with Erikson, J. M., and Kivnick, H. *Vital Involvement in Old Age: The Experience of Old Age in Our Time.* New York: W. W. Norton, 1986.
Foster, Steven. "Passage into Manhood: A Modern Ritual for Young Men." *In Context* 16 (Spring 1987): pp. 50–54.
Gifford-Jones, W. *On Being a Woman: The Modern Woman's Guide to Gynaecology.* New York: Macmillan, 1971.
Giles, Mary, ed. *The Feminist Mystic: And Other Essays on Women and Spirituality.* New York: Crossroad, 1982.
Goldenberg, Naomi. *Changing of the Gods: Feminism and the End of Traditional Religions.* Boston: Beacon Press, 1979.
The Gospel According to Thomas: The Gnostic Sayings of Jesus, trans. Guillaumont et al. New York: Harper & Row, 1984.
Greenwood, Sadja. *Menopause, Naturally: Preparing for the Second Half of Life.* San Francisco: Volcano Press, 1984.
Gross, Rita M. "Suffering, Feminist Theory and Images of Goddess." *Anima* 13, no. 1 (1986): pp. 39–46.
Gutmann, David. *Reclaimed Powers: Towards a New Psychology of Men and Women in Later Life.* New York: Basic Books, 1987.
Hadden, Genia Pauli. *Body Metaphors: Releasing God-feminine in Us All.* New York: Crossroads, 1988.
Harding, Esther. *The Way of All Women.* New York: Harper Colophon, 1970.
————. *Women's Mysteries, Ancient and Modern.* New York: Harper & Row, 1971.
Heilbrun, Carolyn G. *Reinventing Womanhood.* New York: W. W. Norton, 1979.
Huxley, Aldous. *The Perennial Philosophy.* New York: Harper & Row, 1945.
Jacobi, Jolande. *The Way of Individuation.* New York: Harcourt, Brace & World, 1970.
Jung, Carl Gustav. *The Collected Works of C. G. Jung.* Read, Sir H., Fordham, M., and Adler, G., eds., Hull, R.F.C., trans., McGuire, W., exec. ed. Bollingen Series 20, Princeton, NJ: Princeton University Press, 1954.
Johnson, Robert. *Inner Work: Using Dreams and Active Imagination for Personal Growth.* New York: Harper & Row, 1986.
Kaufert, Patricia A., and Gilbert, Penny. "Women, Menopause and Medicalization." *Culture, Medicine & Psychiatry* 10, no. 1 (1986): pp. 7–21.
LeGuin, Ursula. "The Space Crone." *Co-Evolution Quarterly* 10, no. 1 (Summer 1976): pp. 108–111.
Leonard, Linda Schierse. *The Wounded Woman: Healing the Father-Daughter Relationship.* Boulder, CO: Shambhala, 1983.
Lock, Margaret. "Models and Practice in Medicine: Menopause as Symptom or Life Transition?" *Culture, Medicine & Psychiatry* 6 (1982): pp. 261–80.

Mankowitz, Ann. *Change of Life: A Psychological Study of Dreams and the Menopause*. Toronto, Canada: Inner City Books, 1984.

Martin, Emily. *The Woman in the Body: A Cultural Analysis of Reproduction*. Boston: Beacon Press, 1987.

Mead, Margaret. *Male and Female: A Study of the Sexes in a Changing World*. New York: William Morrow, 1949.

Melamed, Elissa. *Mirror, Mirror: The Terror of Not Being Young*. New York: Linden Press, Simon & Schuster, 1983.

Miller, Jean Baker. *Toward a New Psychology of Women*. Boston: Beacon Press, 1976.

Moore, Pat. "Gray Like Me: A Young Woman's Experiment With Aging." *New Age Journal* (March/April 1988).

Morton, Nelle. "The Goddess as Metaphoric Image." Plastow, Judith, and Christ, Carol P., eds. *Weaving the Visions: New Patterns in Feminist Spirituality*. New York: Harper & Row, 1989, pp. 111–18.

Moss, Richard. *The Black Butterfly: An Invitation to Radical Aliveness*. Berkeley, CA: Celestial Arts, 1986.

Neumann, Erich. *The Great Mother: An Analysis of the Archetype*, trans. Ralph Mannheim. Bollingen Series XLVII, Princeton, NJ: Princeton University Press, 1963.

Ornstein, Robert E. *The Psychology of Consciousness*. New York: Penguin, 1972.

Perera, Sylvia Brinton. *Descent to the Goddess: A Way of Initiation for Women*. Toronto, Canada: Inner City Books, 1981.

Perls, Frederick S. *Gestalt Therapy Verbatim*. New York: Bantam, 1970.

Plastow, Judith, and Christ, Carol P., eds. *Weaving the Visions: New Patterns in Feminist Spirituality*. New York: Harper & Row, 1989.

Rich, Adrienne. *Of Woman Born: Motherhood as Experience and Institution*. New York: Bantam, 1977.

Rubin, Lillian. *Women of a Certain Age: The Mid-Life Search for Self*. New York: Harper & Row, 1979.

Scott-Maxwell, Florida. *The Measure of My Days*. New York: Alfred Knopf, 1968.

Shah, Idries. *Learning How to Learn: Psychology and Spirituality in the Sufi Way*. San Francisco: Harper & Row, 1981.

Shuttle, Penelope, and Redgrove, Peter. *The Wise Wound: Eve's Curse and Everywoman: Menstruation as a Powerful and Positive Resource in the Life of Women*. New York: Richard Marek, 1978.

Starhawk. *The Spiral Dance: A Rebirth of the Ancient Religion of the Great Goddess*. San Francisco: Harper & Row, 1979.

Staude, John-Raphael. *Wisdom and Age: The Adventure of Later Life*. Berkeley, CA: Ross Books, 1981.

Stone, Merlin. *When God Was a Woman*. New York: Harvest/HBJ, 1978.

Tavris, Carol, ed. *Everywoman's Emotional Wellbeing, Heart and Mind, Body and Soul*. New York: Doubleday, 1986.

Teish, Luisah. "Ancestor Reverence." Plaskow, Judith, and Christ, Carol, eds.

Weaving the Visions: New Patterns in Feminist Spirituality. San Francisco: Harper & Row, 1989, pp. 87–92.

Trinkaus, E., and Thompson, D. "Femoral Diaphyseal Histomorphometric Age Determinations for the Shanidar 3, 4, 5 & 6 Neandertals and Neandertal Longevity." *American Journal of Physical Anthropology* 72 (1987): pp. 123–29.

Troll, L. E., and Israel, J. K., eds. *Looking Ahead: A Woman's Guide to the Problems and Joys of Growing Older.* Englewood Cliffs, NJ: Prentice-Hall, 1977.

Utian, Wulf. *The Menopause in Modern Perspective: A Guide to Clinical Practice.* New York: Appleton-Century-Crofts, 1980.

————. *Your Middle Years: A Doctor's Guide for Today's Woman.* New York: Appleton-Century-Crofts, 1980.

Van Gennep, Arnold. *The Rites of Passage,* trans. Vizedom, M. B., and Caffee, G. L. Chicago: University of Chicago Press, 1960.

Van Keep, P. A., Utian, W. H., and Vermeulen, A., eds., assisted by Freebody, P. *The Controversial Climacteric.* Workshop moderators' reports presented at the 3rd International Congress on Menopause, held in Ostend, Belgium, under the auspices of the International Menopause Society. Lancaster, England: MTP Press, 1981.

Walker, Barbara. *The Crone: Woman of Age, Wisdom and Power.* New York: Harper & Row, 1985.

Washbourn, Penelope. *Becoming Woman: The Quest for Wholeness in Female Experience.* New York: Harper & Row, 1977.

Weideger, Paula. *Menstruation & Menopause.* New York: Delta, 1977.

Wilbush, Joel. "What's in a Name? Some Linguistic Aspects of the Climacteric." *Maturitas* 3 (1981).

————. "Climacteric Expression & Social Context." *Maturitas* 4 (1982).

INDEX